PSYCHIATRY
IN
GENERAL PRACTICE

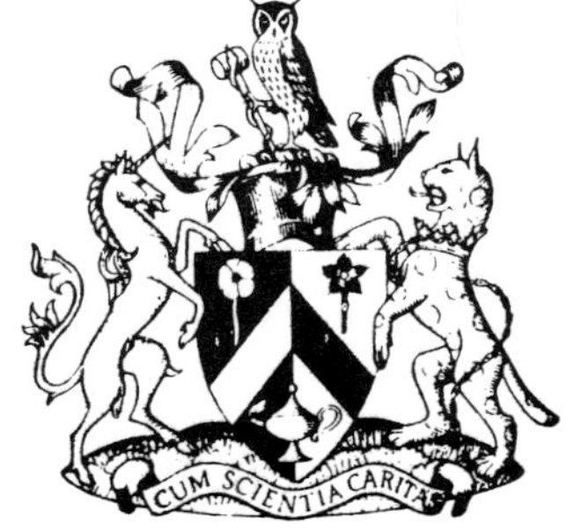

C A H WATTS, OBE, MD, FRCGP, FRCPsych.
and
B M WATTS, MB BS

General Practitioners (retired)
Ibstock, Leicestershire

Published by
The Royal College of General Practitioners

The Royal College of Practitioners was founded in 1952, with this object:

'To encourage, foster, and maintain the highest possible standards in general medical practice and for that purpose to take or join with others in taking steps consistent with the charitable nature of that object which may assist towards the same.'

Among its responsibilities under the Royal Charter the College is entitled to:

'Encourage the publication by general medical practitioners of research into medical or scientific subjects with a view to the improvement of general medical practice in any field and to undertake or assist others in undertaking such research.

Diffuse information on all matters affecting general medical practice and establish, print, publish, issue and circulate such papers, journals, magazines, books, periodicals, and publications and hold such meetings, conferences, seminars, and instructional courses as may assist the object of the College.'

CONTENTS

EDITOR'S PREFACE

1952 was a special year in the history of general practice and will be marked for all time by the establishment of the then College of General Practitioners, later to become Royal in 1967. That event, coming at the mid-point of the 20th century, released for the first time the energies of a vast group of general practitioners. Intellectual stimulation and academic energy have proceeded apace ever since.

Among the Founders of the College were Betty and Arthur Watts, two general practitioners in Ibstock in Leicestershire, and that same year their book, *Psychiatry in General Practice*, was published by J & A Churchill Ltd, one of the leading medical publishers in those days.

The College is republishing this book for several reasons. First, it is an important historical marker, as it is one of the earliest clinical books about general practice written by a general practitioner. It was particularly early – ahead of well-known texts such as John Fry's *The Catarrhal Child* (1961) and *Profiles of Disease* (1967). It therefore stands as an important early text from general practice itself.

Secondly, the clinical content of the book is of both historical and current importance, because the volume of depressive illness at that time is mirrored by the huge load carried by general practitioners today. In 1947, Dr Watts saw 13% of patients as "psychiatric cases", reporting a similar figure in 1950 and 9.9% in 1951 (page 9). Here is the first crucial evidence of the scale of mental and emotional illness in primary care, a finding which was not fully recognised until many years later, when Shepherd *et al.* (1966) in their well-known book, *Psychiatric Illness in General Practice*, confirmed this on a much bigger population.

Because the book was written over forty years ago, there are inevitably words and phrases that are out of date. For instance, there are several references to poorer patients being "on the club" and of course many of the drugs, such as 'Benzedrine' and 'Coramine', are not used at all now.

Moreover, younger practitioners will be quite unfamiliar with wartime phrases such as VADs and Verey lights and may be taken aback by reference to the then illegality of homosexuality and discussion of contraception without mention of the Pill, which had not yet been introduced. There are, however, also phrases that strike a particularly modern note, for example the need to keep drugs "as cheap as possible" (market forces were not unknown even then!). More important are the passages that strike right at the heart of general practice today:

> The vast majority of cases arise from the stresses and strains associated with the home and family life. Indeed a happy home life is the best antidote to most neuroses. The general practitioner is in a unique position to assist in the construction of such homes, if he accepts his responsibility to do so, and in this way he is going far in the direction of prophylactic psychiatry.

Here is some of the encapsulated wisdom accumulated by two general practitioners (it was in fact the theme of the essay for which Betty Watts won the Butterworth Prize) and transmitted across the generations to family doctors today.

Finally, on a topical note, the Royal College of General Practitioners has joined with the Royal College of Psychiatry in the "Defeat Depression Campaign", in order to combat one of the most important chronic illnesses facing general practitioners in the Western world. Here again, Arthur Watts has a special place in history, since his later book, *Depressive Disorders in the Community*, was the first book on this subject from general practice in 1966, and is another classic of its kind. At a time when a major initiative to raise the profile and importance of these diseases in general practice is being undertaken, it seems particularly appropriate that this book should be republished in the College's series of Classic Texts.

Denis Pereira Gray
Honorary Editor

May 1994

FOREWORD

THIS book is written primarily as an introduction to psychiatry in general practice. It is by general practitioners for general practitioners. The authors show what can be done by the family doctor who thinks not alone in terms of organic pathology but also of the dynamics of the patient's mental life. Dr. and Mrs. Watts vividly illustrate in the various case histories which they give, how important it is to recognise psychogenetic factors early in the course of an illness. They also show how relatively straightforward the treatment of the early case can be, and how rewarding such therapy is to the physician.

The topics discussed and the methods employed will, it is hoped, not only excite the reader's interest, but will also encourage him to develop his own personal techniques and skills in this large field of every-day practice. The authors make no claim to have written a text book of psychiatry. What they have done is to provide a comprehensive introduction to psychiatric work as it occurs in general practice. The reader is urged to give their experience and views the full consideration which they merit.

J. D. WYNDHAM PEARCE, MD, FRCPE, DPM
Assistant Physician to the
Department of Psychiatry
St Mary's Hospital, London

Physician
Queen Elizabeth Hospital for Children

PREFACE

"If you are a keen observer of men and things, if you cannot read the book of human nature correctly, and write the
knowledge of physic with an intelligent comprehension of
the thoughts, feelings and desires of mankind, together with
the effects of love, fear, grief, anger, malice, envy, lust and
other stray hidden passions that govern the human race, you
will be sadly deficient even after twenty years' experience."

DE STYRAP, 1889.

This was the advice of an experienced general practitioner
to the young physician 60 years ago. This book is an ampli-
fication of those sentiments made possible by the advances in
psychology which have taken place since he wrote those words.
To the consultant psychiatrist it may appear superficial and
incomplete. It is an attempt to give a bird's eye view of the
problems of psychiatry in general practice.

The clinical material in this book has been collected by one
of us (C.A.H.W.), but because of the pressure of work and
lack of free time in general practice, its presentation in
book form has only been made possible by the co-operation
and assistance of the other (B.M.W.).

Our thanks are extended to all who have helped and en-
couraged us, including Dr. Alice Cox, Dr. W. H. Myburgh,
Dr. J. D. W. Pearce ; and to many friends in the South
African Medical Corps.

Ibstock.

C.A.H.W.
B.M.W.

NOTE ABOUT THE AUTHOR

Dr Arthur Watts OBE, MD, FRCGP, FRCPsych was for many years a general practitioner in Ibstock, Leicestershire. He played a central role in the development of the College of General Practitioners in its early years, keeping with his wife the research register and serving on the Council of the College for several years.

In 1958 he reported the first use of an age-sex register, which developed to be a key tool in helping general practitioners to analyse their practice population and has since become firmly established in general practice throughout the UK.

Having proceeded MD in 1949, Dr Watts went on to achieve many academic distinctions, including the Sir Charles Hastings Prize for Systematic Observation of Research and Record in General Practice awarded by the BMA in 1955, the Hunterian Gold Medal (1957), the James Mackenzie Prize (1971), the Richard Scott Prize (1974), and recently the College's George Abercrombie Award (1993) for his contribution to the literature of general practice.

Dr Watts remained an active supporter of the College throughout his professional lifetime, serving as Provost first of the Midland Faculty and later of the Leicester Faculty.

CHAPTER I

THE PROBLEM

PSYCHIATRY is a subject which interests some people and repels others. Medical men who are attracted to it generally drift into the Mental Hospital Services or consultant practice. Few who are really interested in this subject remain in general practice and those few find themselves, in common with all general practitioners, painfully short of time. The net result appears to be that few general practitioners have either the time or the interest to research into the problem ; and fully trained psychiatrists do not see the type of cases which occur in everyday practice. As a rule only the severe neuroses and frank psychoses are referred to the consultant, and the sphere of work of the trained psychiatrist is largely limited to that type of case. Mild cases and the early stages of mental illness which occur among the ordinary men and women who daily appear in the doctor's surgery are left to develop or clear up on their own. Many are functionally ill, but not ill enough to be passed on to the expert. Here undoubtedly is a wide field for research. This book represents a small excursion into it ; and it is put forward in the hopes of stimulating further exploration by general practitioner workers.

It is usually estimated that one third of the cases seen in general practice are psychological. Statistics taken over four years have shown that here there is an average of 12 per cent of people who are functionally ill, and a further 10 per cent who are suffering from a psychosomatic illness. Exact figures matter little. The point is that a considerable proportion of cases are psychological. These are usually regarded as the bugbear of general practice and the standard treatment is a sedative. Even consultants are guilty of this mode of escapism. All too frequent is the verdict, "I find no signs of organic disease; I have reassured your patient and I suggest she takes pheno. barbitone gr. ½ t.d.s."

There is something seriously wrong with our system of medicine, when a great number of patients who come to us for advice are put off with placebos and are urged out of the surgery with all possible speed, without any attempt at radical treatment.

The reasons for this strange gap in an otherwise fairly efficient and comprehensive system of medicine are threefold.

(i) The average general practitioner and consultant has little knowledge of how to make a differential diagnosis in a psychiatric case. The term "functional" covers everything.

(ii) The current opinion generally is that it takes an expert to perform psychotherapy and it is far beyond the scope of the general practitioner.

(iii) Psychotherapy takes up time, and few practitioners feel they can afford to spend consultation hours with neurotics. The process is looked upon as something magical and mysterious, akin to faith healing and spiritualism, and of doubtful therapeutic value in the end.

These three objections to psychotherapy are worthy of a closer examination.

The Problem of Diagnosis

Few doctors would be satisfied with a diagnosis of cough or anæmia and yet most are quite happy to describe a case as functional. The term "functional" is the label attached to a large waste paper basket into which all these problem cases are deposited. This method of dealing with psychoneurotics is unscientific and wasteful of both patients' and doctors' time.

If on the other hand some reasoned attempt at a differential diagnosis is made, cases can be sorted out and time saved on those which cannot benefit from treatment and expended on those which can; besides which there is considerable satisfaction in a more precise diagnosis.

When a differential diagnosis is made it will be found that cases seen in the surgery fall into one of four categories.

(a) Cases which the general practitioner can treat actively and rationally himself (50 per cent).

(b) Cases which are suffering from a self limiting illness and which need supervision until a natural remission sets in (25 per cent).

(c) Cases which require expert help and advice and must be referred to a psychiatrist (10 per cent).

(d) Cases which are chronic and untreatable by any known methods (15 per cent).

The fourth group is the real waste paper basket but, as can be seen, it forms less than one sixth of all the psychiatric cases.

The Problem of Psychotherapy

There are three grades of surgery. The lowest grade is the work inherited from the barber surgeons, namely, the incision of fluctuating abscesses, the tying off of pedunculated warts and so on. This type of work is a part and parcel of every general practitioner's routine and is performed without question. The second grade of surgery, such as the removal of cysts and simple·tumours and clean minor surgical operations, requires more skill and an aseptic technique, but is still within the scope of any trained medical man. Major surgery is the third grade and it is beyond the scope of the average general practitioner.

In the same way there are three grades of psychotherapy. The first is an essential part of any good doctor's technique, and it consists of seeing the patient against his own background, and appreciating the effect of environment on the patient's condition. The old time general practitioners, living in a more leisurely world, made full use of this technique ; and this to a large extent made up for their lack of the amenities of modern medicine. Doctors who have acquired the habit of building up a strong rapport, and who have won the complete confidence of their patients are in actual fact performing psychotherapy without knowing it, though this treatment is empirical. If a mother is mourning for her child, the sympathetic understanding of the doctor will help her just as much as a bromide mixture.

The second grade of psychotherapy is a reasoned process. It is rational, deeper and more involved than the first grade ; and requires a certain amount of skill and experience ; but like second grade surgery, it is well within the scope of the general practitioner. The patient is worried over some trouble of which he is not fully aware. Neurotic symptoms are evolved to distract the patient's attention from the real problem. The therapist's task is to get behind the smoke screen to discover what is being covered up. The repressed ideas or conflict cause a state of psychological tension or anxiety. Once this tension is released, the bottled up emotions pour out, and the patient feels as relieved as a man who has had a painful tooth removed. The practitioners of old prescribed fox-glove tea for heart disease, a treatment which was effective but empirical. Today we are able to prescribe digitalis with some idea of its action on the conductivity of heart muscle. This is obviously a step forward in therapeutics. In the same way the second grade of psychotherapy is a distinct advance on the old empirical first grade. The latter consists of building up a good rapport and the patient develops such confidence in his doctor that his faith carries him along. The second grade of psychotherapy is an attempt to restore the patient's confidence in himself, to wean him from his doctor, and to make him stand on his own feet.

The third grade of psychotherapy, known as deep therapy, is the province of the specialist. It is a very skilled operation and may take an immense amount of time. It is indeed a major psychiatric operation. When the term psychotherapy is used, doctors and laymen alike frequently think that this deep therapy is implied ; and they fail to realise that there is the minor operation which is successful in the majority of cases which we see in general practice. The psychiatrist also has physical methods for treating some of the more difficult cases, such as electro-convulsive therapy, insulin shock, and leucotomy, but all these are clearly beyond the scope of the general practitioner.

The Problem of Time

The average case requires about four sessions each lasting three quarters of an hour. Thus the *average* time spent on a neurotic is about three hours. Is this too much of one's time in a busy general practice ? In obstetrics I calculate that the time spent on the average case is as follows :—

Description of Attention	Date	Time Taken in Minutes
Booking and General Examination	3rd Month	15
Subsequent A.N. Examination	5th ,,	10
,, ,, ,,	7th ,,	10
,, ,, ,,	8th ,,	10
,, ,, ,,	8½ ,,	10
Confinement	Term	60
5 P.N. Visits Travelling Time Included	Puerperium	50
Final P.N. Examination and Contraceptive Advice	6th Week P.N.	15
TOTAL TIME		180

Thus the amount of time spent on the average obstetric case is about three hours and no conscientious general practitioner would feel the time ill-spent. Few cases are more satisfying than the normal confinement which has gone smoothly according to plan. While the average time is three hours, some cases are "B.B.A." and others take a great deal longer. The same applies to psychotherapy. Some cases can be dealt with efficiently and radically in twenty minutes or half an hour. Others take a good deal longer than the average.

If it is felt that the average time of three hours spent on a functional case is too long, the alternative to radical treatment should be considered. One is saddled with unsatisfied and unsatisfactory patients whose repeated consultations are thoroughly boring. They are frequently loquacious and with weekly consultations at ten minutes a time, the total time spent soon adds up to more than three hours, and in this case they are hours completely wasted, both for the doctor and his patient.

Some of these neurotics become permanent surgery attenders, drawing their certificates week by week or month by month for "nervous debility" or some spurious diagnosis. Some get wearied of inadequate attention and get solace by pouring out their tale of woe to their friends and relations. They waste their money on every quack remedy which promises relief. Some seek other advice by transferring to another practice. Some eventually recover in spite of their doctor, but while the latter may certainly feel relieved at the cessation of their visits, he has long passed the stage at which he might feel much pleasure or satisfaction in their recovery.

The Subconscious Problem. Another deterrent to the practice of psychiatry in general practice lies buried in the subconscious mind, and the objections already enumerated are often rationalisations to cover this real reluctance to use psychiatric methods.

If one compares an acute pneumonia with an acute schizophrenic reaction, one can see one point of comparison and, more obviously, certain great differences. To the man in the street both patients appeared well one day and were seriously ill the next. On the other hand the ætiology of pneumonia is well understood, but the cause of schizophrenia is still wrapped in mystery. It is a problem which baffles the medical man as well as the layman. The patient is profoundly ill and yet there is practically nothing abnormal which either the test tube or the microscope can demonstrate.

From time immemorial mental illness has been taboo and it is surrounded by an aura of mystery which haunts and frightens people. It is for this reason that psychiatry has lagged far behind the other branches of medicine, a point well illustrated by Noel Harris (i). Doctors are human, and the age long spirit of the taboo affects them, just as it affects the layman. Mental illness and nervous illness are not clearly differentiated in the minds of the laity and in many of the medical profession. "A nervous breakdown" is the euphemism used to cover both types of disorder. There is no denying that the newly qualified practitioner is better equipped to diagnose and treat an acute tonsillitis than an anxiety state. The former requires a definite drug, whereas the latter appears to the uninitiated to require a vague mysterious treatment. The aura which surrounds psychiatry depends in part on the gaps in his medical education but also in part in his share of the universal taboo, for all psychiatry is not surrounded by the mystery associated with the frank psychoses. In anxiety states for instance there is a clear cut psychopathology, which, when demonstrated, is as pretty as a smear of blood revealing the parasites of malaria. Psychotherapy in the appropriate case is in fact just as logical as the physical treatment of physical disease.

Psychiatrists themselves are sometimes to blame for the unpopularity of their speciality. Many books on the subject are quite unreadable by the ordinary doctor, so complicated are the theories and so perplexing is the terminology. In many quarters psychiatry is thus regarded as a mass of complex and conflicting ideas wrapped in a jargon of its own and of very little practical value. This belief is furthered by the failure to appreciate that psychiatry at general practice level is very different from that at the consultant level. The former comprises mild cases in their early stages which for the most part respond to simple radical treatment. The latter is composed of the most difficult cases which require deep therapy or complicated treatment. It was of the latter F. P. Haldane (ii) wrote as follows—"The general conclusion surely must be that one or two talks with a psychiatrist are unlikely to effect any very fundamental change in the psycho-neurotic patient. In the end we must put away our lingering hopes of omnipotent thought treatments and recognise that reality requires long and painstaking and difficult work if we wish to treat those who suffer from psycho-neurosis. We must also be still more realistic and realise that at present, apart from a little palliation, many cannot be treated at all."

Any doctor, reading this statement as the opinion of an expert, would certainly be deterred from trying to practise psychotherapy in his surgery. One cannot question this opinion as applied to cases passed on to the specialist in psychiatry, but one can question whether they apply to the majority of cases seen in general practice. Here in the main, the problem is simple; the symptoms are early and with radical treatment the patient can be efficiently and permanently benefited in a few hours. This treatment is the task of the general practitioner and not one for the expert psychiatrist.

Practical Details

The incidence of neuroses and psychoses must vary from place to place and from practitioner to practitioner. Periodically correspondence appears in the press on this subject and figures vary widely from 10 per cent to 60 per cent according to the "outlook and temperament of the doctor himself" (iii).

In order to assess the size of the problem in this practice a series of surveys were made which are analysed below.

Three surveys of 1,000 consecutive cases seen in routine work were made to estimate the proportion of psychiatric cases to other forms of illness ; and an attempt was made to analyse the nature of the psychiatric material by a survey of all functional cases seen over a period of three years. In this latter series no psychosomatic diseases were included but only those which were purely psychiatric. No claim to perfection of diagnosis can be made and the series will no doubt include some errors. However, all recognised mistakes have been excluded. The figures should be regarded as a rough guide to the incidence of psychiatric illness, compiled as they were during the surgery hours of a fairly busy practice. They give a useful bird's-eye view of the actual numbers and type of cases which confront the general practitioner.

SURVEYS OF 1000 CONSECUTIVE CASES

	Sept.-Nov. 1947		June-July 1950		Jan.-Feb. 1951	
	No. of Cases	Total	No. of Cases	Total	No. of Cases	Total
MEDICAL CASES						
Gastro-intestinal diseases	127		131		65	
Respiratory diseases .	139		94		178	
Skin diseases . .	53		64		44	
Infectious diseases .	47		51		238	
Rheumatic diseases .	45		50		55	
Heart diseases . .	22		31		18	
Nervous diseases . .	21		23		24	
Diseases peculiar to children . . .	27		11		10	
Neurovascular diseases .	17		16		14	
Genito urinary diseases .	16		15		12	
Blood diseases . .	10		17		9	
Metabolic diseases .	8	532	10	513	8	675
SURGICAL CASES						
Trauma . . .	128		97		59	
General surgical . .	48		70		42	
E.N.T. diseases . .	50		65		55	
Eye diseases . .	22	248	37	269	17	173
GYNÆCOLOGY AND OBSTETRICS						
Obstetrics . . .	38		46		33	
Gynæcology . . .	34	72	25	71	10	43
PSYCHIATRIC CASES . .	133	133	134	134	99	99
ADMINISTRATIVE CASES .	15	15	13	13	10	10
		1000		1000		1000

Two of these surveys were performed when the practice was comparatively slack. With the advent of winter and spring epidemics the percentage of psychiatric illness falls in comparison with other complaints, as is shown in the Jan.-Feb. survey.

The cases in the three year survey were divided into acute and chronic. It will be noted that the number of new chronic cases falls rapidly in each successive year ; but unfortunately those first seen in 1948 are for the most part still constant attenders in 1950. They are the incurables, but they form only 14.5 per cent of the total.

These tables show that during the period under review a grand total of 670 psychiatric cases were seen of which 97 were chronic and largely unsuitable for treatment. Nine in the series were referred from outside the practice, and four of these were schizophrenics. Only one referred case was suitable for treatment at general practice level. 59 cases were referred to a psychiatrist, but of these 13 refused to go. Of the 46 who sought specialist advice, 24 were admitted to a mental

THREE YEAR SURVEY

ACUTE CASES					
	1948	1949	1950	Total	Average
Anxiety states:					
Generalised anxiety .	20	23	19	62	21
Somatic dysfunction.	42	28	52	122	41
Depressed type .	29	20	32	81	27
Phobic type . .	26	10	19	55	18
Children under 15 .	19	18	17	54	18
Total .	136	99	139	374	125
Endogenous depression	52	47	44	143	48
Hysteria:					
Hystero-anxiety .	8	9	5	22	7
Frank hysteria. .	8	6	5	19	6
Total .	16	15	10	41	14
Schizophrenia . .	5	2	1	8	3
Mania . . .			1	1	0·3
Compensation neurosis.	3	2	1	6	2
Total .	212	165	196	573	192

<table>
<tr><td colspan="6" align="center">CHRONIC CASES</td></tr>
<tr><td></td><td>1943</td><td>1249</td><td>1950</td><td>Total</td><td>Average</td></tr>
<tr><td>Anxiety states . .</td><td>25</td><td>13</td><td>3</td><td>41</td><td>14</td></tr>
<tr><td>Endogenous depression</td><td>16</td><td>3</td><td>1</td><td>20</td><td>7</td></tr>
<tr><td>Hypochondiasis with mental defect . .</td><td>6</td><td>3</td><td>2</td><td>11</td><td>4</td></tr>
<tr><td>Psychopathic personality . . . .</td><td>4</td><td>2</td><td>2</td><td>8</td><td>3</td></tr>
<tr><td>Obsessional neurosis .</td><td>2</td><td>—</td><td>—</td><td>2</td><td>0·6</td></tr>
<tr><td>Schizophrenia . .</td><td>—</td><td>1</td><td>2</td><td>3</td><td>1·0</td></tr>
<tr><td>Mania . . .</td><td>1</td><td>1</td><td>—</td><td>2</td><td>0·6</td></tr>
<tr><td>Paranoia . . .</td><td>—</td><td>1</td><td>—</td><td>1</td><td>0·3</td></tr>
<tr><td>Paraphrenia . .</td><td>—</td><td>—</td><td>1</td><td>1</td><td>0·3</td></tr>
<tr><td>Mental defect . .</td><td>—</td><td>2</td><td>2</td><td>4</td><td>1·3</td></tr>
<tr><td>Alcoholic psychosis .</td><td>—</td><td>1</td><td>1</td><td>2</td><td>0·6</td></tr>
<tr><td>Senile psychosis . .</td><td>—</td><td>—</td><td>2</td><td>2</td><td>0·6</td></tr>
<tr><td align="center">Total . . .</td><td>54</td><td>27</td><td>16</td><td>97</td><td></td></tr>
</table>

hospital for treatment. Only two are still in hospital and are likely to stay there, and a further two will probably end their days in an institution but at present their relations are putting up with them at home. In three years of 142 acute depressions only one has committed suicide.

No recovery rate was worked out in this series of patients but, by applying figures from collateral series, an approximate figure can be assessed.

CASES TREATABLE IN GENERAL PRACTICE

	RECOVERY	IMPROVED	I.S.Q.
Anxiety states, etc.	40%	38%	22%
Endogenous depression.	61%	15%	24%
Average Total.	50·5%	26·5%	23%

From this it can be seen that with proper handling 50·5 per cent of suitable psychiatric cases can be expected to recover completely and cease to be a burden on the general practitioner. In all some 77 per cent derive benefit from such treatment and about 23 per cent are referred to a specialist, drift away or sink into a chronic psychiatric state.

There is one more important aspect of this problem. This practice consists of about 8,000 people, and from these every year more than 200 new cases of psychiatric illness are seen. If the same incidence obtains over the whole country, there must be some 1,200,000 fresh psychiatric cases occurring each year out of our population of 48,000,000 people. This figure is only a very rough gauge of the problem, but it shows its immensity. It is obviously quite beyond the scope of the psychiatric services to deal with such numbers, which do *not* include all the chronic sick. If the problem is going to be tackled at all, the brunt of the burden must fall on the general practitioner. He has to bear it in any case, but it is easier to bear if treated honestly and rationally, instead of empirically with sedative and placebo.

In most branches of medicine, the specialist has certain considerable advantages over the general practitioner. He has at his service all the manifold methods of investigation which are often denied to those in general practice. He has wider scope for investigation and more accurate methods of clinching the diagnosis. In psychiatry, the position is reversed. The general practitioner has certain advantages over the specialist. Living among his patients, he knows many of them before they are ill and so has a more accurate norm with which to compare his patient. He knows the background against which the patient lives his life. He knows his family and his family history often without making any inquiries. In a psychiatric interview the consultant gets as it were only a cross section of the patient's life. The general practitioner has in addition the longitudinal section, which can only be obtained by the psychiatrist after a period of observation.

The consultant has only very few diagnostic weapons which are not available to the general practitioner.

During the past 50 years so much of our demesne has been taken away from us that there is a danger that we may become finger posts directing our patients to the most appropriate specialist. We no longer set our own fractures, or even treat our own fevers or tuberculosis. We are being driven out of the hospitals, and in general our work in one way or another is being curtailed and limited. Here in psychiatry is a new sphere of work for our attention. It is essentially work for general practitioners and a more rational outlook on the problem is long overdue.

REFERENCES

(i) NOEL G. HARRIS. Modern Trends in Psychological Medicine. 1948.
(ii) F. P. HALDANE. *Lancet* 1950 (1) p. 793.
(iii) H. BOLTON TIPLER. *B.M.J.* 1948 (1) p. 570.

CHAPTER II

THE MECHANISM OF ANXIETY

Definition

It can be seen from the statistics in the previous chapter that roughly half (56 per cent) of all psychiatric cases seen in general practice are anxiety states. The treatment of these cases is therefore the main part of the psychiatric problem confronting the general practitioner, and with proper handling most of them recover or at least improve.

An anxiety state is described by Ross (i) as "a series of symptoms which arise from a faulty adaptation to the stresses and strain of life". Thus the anxiety state is a form of stress disease, indeed the commonest manifestation of that problem. Peptic ulcer, hypertension and osteo-arthritis are all recognised today as due to failure of the general adaptation syndrome. Some of these diseases have been traced back to earlier stages. In the ulcer syndrome, nervous dyspepsia is certainly the forerunner of ulcer formation. Anxiety precedes the nervous dyspepsia and it is logical to assume that adequate treatment of anxiety in its early stages may prevent later stages arising before these conditions have become established and perhaps irreversible. When one considers the working time lost and suffering endured through these diseases, it is obviously socially economical and humane to attempt treatment in the very earliest stages.

The definition of anxiety state may be illustrated by a very simple example of the sort of case likely to be seen by a general practitioner. J.B., a girl of 18, came to see me complaining of a pain in her left upper arm. I could find no evidence of organic disease. I told her I could find no physical explanation of the pain but that pains of this nature were very often nervous in origin. I told her that worry could cause pain, and before I could say any more she asked me to tell her something about cancer. When I asked her why she wanted to know about it, she told me that three weeks previously she had bumped her left breast and she thought there was a lump there. She had heard that this was how cancer started. I examined the breast but there was no evidence of a lump. I showed her how, by pinching the breast tissue, one could feel a spurious lump. I was able thoroughly to reassure her. She came to report two weeks later and all her troubles had gone. The treatment took about 20 minutes in all.

In this very simple case the mechanism is typical. She thought she had a cancer, but the thought was so terrifying that she tried hard to repress the idea and when her anxiety was expressed as a pain in the arm, she concentrated her attention on it. Very few neurotics come straight to the point. The presenting symptom is almost invariably something which they find easier to talk and think about than their real fear. By concentrating on the symptom the original fear is in fact repressed and may be completely forgotten. In this patient the whole psychopathology lay above the conscious level, and it was easy to explain the whole case and put the blame where it rightly belonged. The trouble was cleared in one short session. It would have been quicker to call the pain "muscular rheumatism" and to have prescribed various placebos, but this is neither scientific nor honest and might well have prolonged the condition by making the girl believe there really was something wrong. She might have been told that I could find nothing wrong with her arm, and I could simply have reassured her by saying she had nothing to worry about. In practice such reassurance rarely works. The patient feels snubbed, as the only logical conclusion is that the doctor is implying that the pain is imaginary or that she is "putting it on". We have all met patients who start their tale with the preamble "I have been to several other doctors and they all say there is nothing the matter with me, but I cannot convince myself that they are right". The only line to take is to accept the fact of the pain and to discover an adequate cause for it. By uncovering the fear of cancer in this case I exposed the real trouble, and by discussing the problem logically I cleared the symptoms rapidly without any placebo or further treatment.

The Natural History of Anxiety

Nature has endowed the more primitive creatures with instinctive reactions which protect the animal from the most obvious stresses and strains. Hunger sends the lion out to seek its prey. Shortening days and colder weather warn the swallows to congregate in preparation for migration to warmer climates. The fear reaction is a very quick and powerful mechanism. In Africa I came across the cub of some wild cat. It was so young it could hardly walk, but it was so well protected with tooth and claw and a powerful fear reaction that I could not get near it without risking severe scratches and bites.

The reactions of our primitive ancestors would also be comparatively simple. Their everyday problems would be few, such as the search for food and shelter, the quest of a mate and the necessity of finding protection from other men and wild beasts. With the evolution of property, live stock and, in the end, cultivated land, man's environment became more and more complicated, and more subject to stress and strain. As intelligence progressed, imagination came into being. Animals live entirely in the present, but man developed the additional capacity of living in the past and fearing for the future. The cat develops a fear reaction only when it hears, sees, or smells a dog approaching. The human being can fear a lion or a burglar which does not really exist. Fear in an animal is largely a passing incident. Fear in man may become a semi-permanent state of mind. An elderly woman heard strange noises in the night and the next morning discovered that the lock-up shop next door had been burgled. For weeks afterwards any noise in the night meant burglars to her, and she was unable to sleep because of her fears. She knew these fears were irrational, as no burglar would want to steal from her humble home and in any case she had her husband sleeping beside her to protect her, but her fears persisted.

Anxiety is a process of fear prolonged in time. The fear reaction, with its fight or flight response, is the outcome of sympathetic stimulation of the adrenals. Anxiety produces a state of chronic emotional tension, which, by way of the autonomic nervous system and the endocrines, produces the manifold somatic manifestations associated with anxiety states.

In the early stages of a neurosis the anxiety is free. The patient feels vaguely unwell, tensed up and without any clear cut symptoms. The threshold for noxious stimuli is lowered. A headache that would normally be treated by an aspirin and forgotten becomes an evil omen and persists. Any symptom tends to produce more anxiety, and anxiety itself tends to exaggerate the symptom so that a vicious circle is formed. Sooner or later the free anxiety crystallises into a set of symptoms which may collect round some organ of the body, or be expressed as a phobia or depression. The increased tension causes an increase in muscle tone, so that the reflexes become exaggerated. Individual muscles or muscle groups may be put into spasm which produce pain. The pain of a neurotic is not imaginary. It is as real as any toothache, and is often caused by this muscle spasm. The more observant patients sometimes notice this. One young man with effort syndrome complained of pain "over his heart" and he noticed that when the pain was on, his left pectoralis muscles were hard and tender to touch.

The Nature of Adverse Circumstances

It was suggested earlier that the environmental strain which confronted our ancestors was much more simple than the stress of life today. Actually there are big changes even in the last fifty years. The tempo of life is faster and the world is smaller. A war in China today affects our lives, whereas in those days the Far East was a world apart. Bad news can reach us quickly from all quarters of the globe. We risk our lives every time we cross a road. In the leisurely days which closed the nineteenth century few of our modern tensions existed, but today, when life is so insecure and arduous for many people, there is an almost infinite variety of factors which may give rise to strain and anxiety.

The *exciting causes* of anxiety states seen were analysed and the adverse factors could be grouped under four main headings :

A.	Frustration	45 per cent
B.	Insecurity	35 per cent
C.	Sexual problems	16 per cent
D.	Guilt feelings	4 per cent

Frustration in one form or other was the commonest cause of anxiety states. Unsuitable or unsatisfying work was common, and so was the wearisome problem of married couples living in rooms or with relations. The acute emotional upsets of a broken courtship were surprisingly rare. In one-third of the cases frustration was due to friction in the home, and in half these marriage problems the breach was serious but in half it was trivial and easily remedied.

Insecurity was the usual basis of childhood neuroses, but it also played a big part in the production of adult anxiety states. When a new baby arrived and an older child was deposed, there was often an anxiety reaction expressed in some behaviour problem. In adult life insecurity might arise from fear of a disease. Very occasionally this reaction was understandable and inevitable. I saw two cousins who were descended from a family tainted with Hur ington's chorea. Forty was the usual age at which the symptoms of this hopeless disease developed, and as they approached this age they became worried and anxious. Quite frequently a similar reaction was based on an entirely erroneous diagnosis of heart disease in youth which had undermined the patient's confidence in himself. The insecurity factor played a part in the anxiety of people who had had an unhappy childhood with quarrelsome parents, or who had been born "on the wrong side of the blanket". A large group were over-attached to one or other parent, usually the mother. Death of this parent or separation from her by leaving home or marriage, with a resultant feeling of insecurity, became the precipitating cause of the anxiety state. Similarly compensation neurosis in some cases arose from a sense of insecurity. The patient did not dare to relinquish his pension on which he lived a frugal existence, in case he was unable to work in open competition.

Sexual Problems. These problems commonly arose from sexual immaturity derived from ignorance in these matters and a consequent unhappy start to married life. Disappointment over sterility was not uncommon, or its opposite, the fear of pregnancy. Homosexuality was rare ; and the problems of masturbation and puberty were surprisingly uncommon.

Feelings of Guilt. Feelings of guilt occurred mainly as a venereal disease phobia. In the army guilt feelings were common among soldiers who had become "bomb happy" and who felt that they had failed as soldiers to live up to their own ideals.

Levels of Consciousness

Confronted with an unsatisfactory situation a man can be aware of his difficulties at different levels of consciousness. He may be completely aware of the real difficulty ; or he may rationalise, that is, he may blame other factors which really have nothing to do with the actual case. Most volunteers in an army would claim patriotism as the motive which had made them join up. Actually this is a rare incentive. Some seek adventure, others are glad to escape from a nagging wife or a monotonous job, and others are driven by the herd instinct to don khaki like the rest. Sometimes the real problem is completely buried in the unconscious mind. It may be just below the level of consciousness, or it may be very deep down. The nearer to the conscious level a memory lies, the easier the treatment and the converse is of course, equally true.

If a man loses his mother he is depressed and sad. His efficiency is impaired and he may even weep. There is no need to tell him why he is depressed; he is perfectly conscious of the cause. The normal individual should be able to meet such a situation with a minimal impairment of efficiency and he should be more or less adjusted to life again in two weeks. If he is so prostrated with grief as to fail to return to normal in that time there is probably an additional cause for his depression, a cause which lies hidden below the level of consciousness. In other words his depression is not due only to the conscious sense of separation from his mother, but there are other factors of which he is unaware. He may feel he could have done more for his mother when she was alive, or that her death was hastened by some failure of his, and he transfers his sorrow at his failure, to his original overt sorrow. In one case the mother died of meningitis. The family said it was due to a shock, and the patient always felt some trivial misdeed of his had given her that shock; his remorse and fear at this idea was transformed and added to his grief. He may be subconsciously glad she has gone ; but such an idea is so repugnant to the conscious mind that it is deeply repressed and heavily disguised by a picture of overwhelming grief.

When the patient fails to correlate his symptoms with the true cause of his anxiety, or when the problem lies buried in the unconscious, the picture becomes one of an anxiety state. In such a condition the patient concentrates all his attention on his symptoms thereby avoiding the real issue, and the real problem is evaded or forgotten.

Types of Anxiety State

While the basic psychopathology of all anxiety states is similar, the variety of the symptoms is such as to make it advisable to describe various types of the condition. These are as follows :—

16·5%   (A) Free anxiety in which no clear symptoms are defined.

32·6% (B) Anxiety states with somatic dysfunction, effort syndrome, nervous dyspepsia, etc.

21·6% (C) Anxiety states with depressive symptoms. This condition has various names such as re-active, exogenous, or secondary depression.

14·8% (D) Anxiety states with phobic symptoms, such as venereal disease phobia : claustrophobia, etc.

14·5% (E) *Childhood neuroses are often expressed as behaviour problems or mannerisms and tics.

The various types of anxiety state and their mechanisms can best be illustrated by case histories.

Mrs. A.M. (37). This is a simple case of free unattached anxiety in which the problem lay at conscious level. The patient was merely failing to correlate her symptoms with her circumstances. The treatment took up an hour, and the patient recovered completely.

Mrs. A.M. came to see me because she had felt vaguely unwell and depressed for about six months. She was given to crying and could not sleep at nights. She said she was just run down and wanted a tonic. The background was as follows. She had two children and was expecting a third. She was look-ing forward to the new baby. Her home was in Coventry but after the destruction of the city she had evacuated to the country. She was fortunate enough to find a rather squalid cottage which she did not have to share. Towards the end of 1945 she applied for a new house in her home town among her own people. After the usual delays she was informed that as she already had a house, she was ineligible for a house in Coventry. This letter precipitated her anxiety state. In addition she was lonely as her husband was still in the forces. She was at a disadvantage being pregnant, and she felt gener-ally frustrated and could see no way of getting back to normal life. She felt better after she had told me of her troubles, and the promise of a letter to the authorities encouraged her. My letter bore fruit and three months later she moved back to

*See later chapter.

Coventry. She wrote to me after the birth of her third son, and told me she had never felt better in her life.

This was a very mild anxiety state amounting to no more than the obvious reaction to frustration. She came to me for a tonic, but there is no medicine which will cure frustration. I pointed out that her feelings of "unwellness" were due to adverse circumstances, and I made her place the blame rationally where it belonged. My letter to the authorities helped in a very practical way by removing the frustration completely.

Mr. B.J. (45). This is a more complicated case of an anxiety state with depressive features. The problem lay at the conscious level, but the patient had rationalised his troubles, and was blaming the wrong things. The case took up three hours of my time.

B.J. was a deputy at the pit. He came to see me because his nerves were in a bad way and he could not sleep at night. He was finding his work a strain and he felt he was losing his grip of his job and the men under him. He felt all the time "something awful" was going to happen. The telephone ringing where he was on duty sent him into a panic, as he felt it meant an accident or bad news. He was so depressed he wept as he told me about himself.

He had lost his wife from cancer two years previously and life, with three sons to care for, had been difficult for him. For a year before her death he had known the diagnosis, but had kept it to himself. His family, who had never approved of his marriage, were very offhand and unsympathetic about his troubles. They had never once visited his wife during her illness. With encouragement he told me in a hesitant manner of yet another problem. His eldest son, a lad of eighteen, had put an undesirable girl in a family way. What hurt him most about it was that he had heard the news from the girl's father. He blamed himself for this as he felt he must have lost the boy's confidence. In the course of discussion it became clear that he had been losing his grip, not of his men at work, but of his family at home. Gradually he regained confidence in himself, and on his own accord he talked things over with his son again. In the final session he told me that they had made up their minds on a plan of action and they would do it "together". He was off work for three weeks, but I haven't seen him as a patient for the past three years. At the beginning of the treatment he was depressed enough to cry in public. He blamed his work, but this was only a rationalisation of his home worries. Once these problems were boldly faced up to, his depression left him.

Pte. A.B. (24). This is a more complicated case of an anxiety state with somatic dysfunction. He was actually a case of effort syndrome. The precipitating psychiatric trauma lay below the level of consciousness. The case took six hours and he was much improved by the treatment before leaving hospital but as he was a military case no follow up was possible.

The patient complained of what he called "Heart attacks". These he described as a feeling of terror. His heart began to pound, he felt a tight band round his chest, and he could not get his breath. He was quite sure he would die in one of these attacks and he felt they were sometimes precipitated by drinking beer. It always had a bad effect on him. His first attack had come on while boarding a train to go on leave to his wife. He had managed to get on to a carriage seat but for half an hour he did not know whether he would live or die, he felt so ill. When I asked him where beer came into the picture, he told me that he and his friends had flung a party the night before. He admitted he had been drunk for the first time in his life. He had been strictly brought up and his parents were both staunch temperance people. He had quite a conscience on the matter of taking alcohol in any form, and he dare not let his people know how he had fallen from grace. While we were discussing the matter of intoxicants, he suddenly stopped talking. "I have just remembered something I never told you." I encouraged him to talk and he said he wasn't sure whether it was reality or a dream, he was too drunk to be certain ; but it was just faintly possible that at this party he had seduced one of the A.T.S. girls present! He tried to minimise the admission by hoping that it was a dream : but it was clear beyond all doubt that he had in fact been unfaithful to his wife. He had successfully repressed this unhappy incident and forgotten all about it. His conscience worked underground, and the normal feelings of remorse were replaced by the symptoms of his so called heart attack. He was able to go back to his wife feeling sorry for himself instead of suffering from his seared conscience. She was able to make the bargain even more profitable by sympathising with him. Had she known the truth her reactions would have been very different.

To understand why his symptoms took the form they did one had to go further back in his life.

In the Western Desert he had found air attacks very trying, On one occasion as he lay in his slit trench, the machine gun bullets came so close to him that they spurted sand over him. He had hardly recovered from this alarm when Stukas arrived. He could bear it no longer. He ran headlong across the desert in a complete panic, until he could run no further. He dropped into an empty slit trench and lay there until his comrades came for him. He was all in. He knew he was "yellow" and could not face them. He was repatriated shortly afterwards. This unpleasant memory was wholly conscious. Under the strain of air attack he had gone into a panic, and this reaction had filled him with remorse. Thus in his mind panic and guilt were associated. Eighteen months later his conscience was again damaged, this time by his infidelity. On this occasion the incident was successfully repressed but while guilt was obscured, panic took its place. His symptoms were a "feeling of panic sweeps over me : my pulse starts racing, there is a tight band round my chest and I cannot get my breath". He must have felt like that when he fell exhausted into the slit trench.

To summarise the pathology of this case ; the symptoms were those of effort syndrome. The cause of the neurosis was the repression of a memory loaded with guilt. The form of the neurosis was conditioned by a previous experience of panic which was also associated with guilt. The purpose of the neurosis was to escape the memory of an unthinkable act he had performed while drunk. The bargain with himself was useful at first. It made the reunion with his wife congenial, but the bargain was a bad one in the end, as he went in fear of his life.

Miss M.C. (38). This case was an anxiety state with phobic symptoms. The patient was a nurse who feared she was poisoning her patients, and, though she knew her fears were irrational, she was quite unable to evade them. The neurosis was profound and had its origin in childhood and was associated with memories and experiences deeply repressed. The patient was seen three times a week for three months.* The result was an improvement though she could not be counted as a recovery. It is however an interesting example of a phobia in an anxiety state and demonstrates the part that childhood experiences can play in adult reactions.

Miss M.C. was a nurse aged 38 years, who had suffered somewhat grieviously at the hands of the medical profession. At 36 she had an attack of renal colic. She was fully investigated and X-rayed from every angle. After six weeks of this the senior surgeon told her that the investigations showed that she had a hypernephroma with secondaries in the lungs and that nothing could be done about it. Up to this point she had never felt really ill, and the diagnosis was a great surprise and shock to her. When she had had time to consider the verdict she asked for another opinion. She was transferred to a different hospital and all the investigations were repeated. At the end she was told that her kidneys were completely exonerated but that the lung shadows remained and were presumably tubercular. She was therefore treated as a consumptive for some weeks but as the shadows did not change it was decided that the lesions must have healed. She was allowed to get up and after some sick leave she returned to work in the hospital. It was then phobia began to develop.

---

*This case was dealt with under hospital conditions, and because of the time factor would be unsuitable for treatment in general practice.

She became uncertain about handing out medicine to her patients. She had a horror of poisoning them. She would pour out half an ounce of cough medicine, but before she reached her patient she felt perhaps it was the wrong medicine or perhaps she had measured too much. The dose would be poured down the drain and she would start afresh. If the medicine ever got as far as the patient she suffered hours of mental agony wondering if he would survive.

She reported her troubles to her medical officer who diagnosed thyrotoxicosis, but a normal B.M.R. soon ruled that out. She was referred to another physician who diagnosed amœbiasis but a course of emetine proved ineffective. Then, as so often happens in these cases, the issue was evaded completely and she was made home sister. Her duties kept her out of the wards and she supervised the nurses' quarters and feeding. All went well for a few months and then she found herself getting suspicious about the food. She kept tasting the various dishes and if they were not to her liking they were thrown out as suspect. Innocent tins of condensed milk and other foods found their way into the dustbin because of her fear of poisoning people and finally she had to give up her post. It was at this stage she came under my care.

Her psychiatric history showed very briefly that she had been over-attached to her father. She had had two offers of marriage but had turned down both of her suitors because they did not, to her mind, compare favourably with her father. Her mother died of cancer at the age of 36 when the patient was a child of 12. She remembered her mother's illness and how night after night, she had dreamed of her mother's death. When her mother finally did die, she told her aunt who came to break the news to her that she had dreamed it in the night and she was accepted in the family as having second sight. When I enquired how often she had dreamed of her mother after that, she could remember no dreams at all and I concluded that her dreams were a death wish. She wanted her mother out of the way so that she could possess her father completely.

After her mother's death, her mother's sister came to keep house and for two years all went well. Then the father married the aunt. The patient was furious beyond description. She refused to attend the wedding and was as unpleasant as a girl of 14 could be. Her resentment over this matter was still evident. She referred to her step-mother as "mother" when speaking to people outside the family as that prevented questions being asked, but she insisted on addressing her to her face as "aunt". She did not mind her as an aunt but refused to accept her as a mother substitute.

This brief sketch of the background gives an indication of the psychopathology. She was firmly fixated to her father and she wished her mother to die. When this occurred, she was 12 years old and she felt subconsciously well satisfied at the removal of her rival. The mother died of cancer at the age of 36. At the self-same age the patient was threatened with death from the same disease—an appropriate punishment for such an evil daughter. She was reprieved in the end, but the death wish which had lain dormant for so long now produced a conscience reaction expressed in the phobia. Having escaped just retribution for wishing her mother dead, she was determined to be responsible for no one else's life.

When she first began to see this explanation for her phobia she was loath to accept it but in the intervals between sessions she recalled and was haunted by an early memory that persuaded her that the mechanism was reasonable. As a very small girl she remembered her father singing while her mother played the piano and the very great pleasure she derived from a song in which the mother died and father and daughter were left all in all to each other.

The end result of this case is not known as I lost contact with her owing to Army transfers, at a time when she had been able to resume work and was pleased to find that she could now hand out aspirins to her patients without qualms.

These cases have been used as examples to illustrate the four main types of symptoms appearing in anxiety states.

It must be admitted, however, that some cases do not fall neatly into any one class and many cases are mixed. It is possible for a depressed patient to have a phobia or to develop a nervous dyspepsia ; but while the presenting picture in an anxiety state can be very variable, the psychopathology and treatment follow roughly the same lines in each case. Adverse circumstances have given rise to anxiety and there are two obvious methods of relieving the situation, namely to change the patient's reaction or to change the circumstances.

In the first place an attempt should be made to make the patient face up to the problem openly and honestly. If psychotherapy is insufficient to alter the patient's attitude and behaviour, then, if possible the circumstances must be altered to suit the patient. Sometimes neither of these courses is possible and then the treatment fails. Psychotherapy is no cure all. There are plenty of medical and surgical cases for which we have at present no remedy and the only course is to make the best attempt we can to alleviate the symptoms.

What happens to the neurotic who is left to fend for himself, aided perhaps by some sedative from the doctor ? Some undoubtedly recover on their own. Circumstances causing the anxiety may alter, and so change the picture. Unfortunately if a patient has been anxious long enough the conditions may become chronic so that even when the circumstances are changed for the better, he remains neurotic and is well on the road to becoming a hypochondriac. Some learn to live with their symptoms, and carry on in spite of them. As time passes they are reassured and ultimately the dread passes off, but it is often a long and wearisome process, compared to the rapid recovery following psychotherapy. They remain anxiety prone, and more liable than the average person to fall a victim to anxiety should new stresses arise in life. A few actually cure themselves. One patient of 50 told me that as a young man in the twenties, he was convinced he had a bad heart. He was apprehensive about himself, and life was a burden to him. Reassurance from his doctor never convinced him. One day as he drove some cattle to a neighbouring village he decided to satisfy himself, or die in the attempt. Having disposed of his charges, he ran the three miles home across the fields. Much to his pleasure and surprise he was none the worse for his exertion and his heart fear faded out never to return.

Many cases become chronic, and their fears and symptoms persist through life. It is often suggested that people over 35 are poor subjects for psychotherapy. Their minds have lost the flexibility of youth and cannot cope with the treatment. While this is usually the case, it is not a universal rule. One woman patient of mine, aged 48, came to see me complaining of nocturnal eneuresis of life long duration; 4 or 5 times a week she wet the bed, and in spite of her husband's tactful tolerance she was miserable about it. In spite of her age, psychotherapy has now reduced these accidents to rare occurrences averaging once a month, and when they do occur she is not very upset. I am disappointed not to be able to free her entirely of this symptom but she herself is well satisfied. She says she is better than she has been for years in every way, and of her own initiative took a holiday last year, a thing she had never dared to do before.

However, it is true with psychotherapy as in all medicine, the earlier a problem is tackled the better the prognosis and many neglected neurotics become hypochondriacs living a miserable life with innumerable symptoms for which one can find no cause and no cure. Socially they are a major problem, as many working days are lost and many a family unit is rendered unstable and unhappy. Anxiety is not transmitted in the genes as many patients imagine ; but anxious parents do rear anxious children. This is another very good reason for treating all young neurotics, so that they may be prevented from becoming dangerously anxious parents.

When I was being introduced to psychiatry in the army many of my colleagues had a pessimistic view of the subject. "Once a neurotic, always a neurotic" was a catch phrase, and some suggested that once you had undertaken psychotherapy, you would have your patient round your neck (or on your doorstep) ever more. In the army one could hardly form a judgment on this matter as patients were transferred away and disappeared from sight. In general practice one lives among one's patients all the time. I find it quite exceptional to have a treated case causing embarrassment by returning again and again for advice or reassurance. There are still some incurables, but far fewer than there would have been without psychotherapy.

REFERENCE

(i) T. A. Ross. The Common Neuroses. 1937.

CHAPTER III

PRACTICAL MEASURES

Introduction

So far we have been concerned with the incidence of psychiatric illness in general practice ; and the mechanism of anxiety states has been described in some detail. Before treatment is started a diagnosis must obviously be made.

A psychiatric diagnosis is not based on physical signs, as in general medicine, but on symptoms, and what may be termed "the feel of the case". The practical physician who is used to having his diagnosis of tuberculosis confirmed beyond all doubt by a positive sputum test or cavity shadows in the X-ray plates feels perhaps that he is abandoning firm ground and stepping into a morass of uncertainty, if he is to depend on these two factors : and yet even the most practical is in the habit of separating out his functional from his organic cases, by just this means. He is influenced not only by the fact that the patient's symptoms do not fit in with any organic lesion, but also by the manner and bearing of the patient, who is unduly worried about himself and pressing about a diagnosis. Very early in a medical career, one learns that the patient who says "I have a pain in my chest ; what causes it?" is different from, and more difficult than the patient who merely states his symptoms. It does not take very long for any doctor to become fairly confident in diagnosing his functional cases from the character of their symptoms, their attitude, and the "feel of the case". To differentiate between the various types of psychiatric illness a similar process is used. Let us take a few obvious examples. One may not approve of alcoholic intoxication, but the man who is "happy" can, and often does, make his audience happy too. His forth-right remarks and his good humour amuse and infect his companions with good cheer. Much the same applies to the maniac patient who brings with him an aura of hearty congeniality. On the other hand the depressed patient is depressing and makes one feel sad. As experience in psychiatric medicine increases, the use one makes of this instrument of diagnosis, increases one's sensitivity and powers of judgment. To begin with one is guided largely by symptoms. Later it is by the patient's reaction to treatment and the feel of the case, that one makes the diagnosis. This comes into play especially when the diagnosis is more difficult. One is guided not so much by what the patient says but by his attitude and his actions. Freud gives a very clear picture of this process. "He that hath eyes to see and ears to hear may convince himself that no mortal can keep a secret. If his lips are silent he chatters with his finger tips, and betrayal oozes out of him from every pore" (i).

In this chapter the general approach to any functional case is described in some detail, leading on to the treatment of anxiety states in particular. First a very simple line of approach is described in which any general practitioner can make a start, so that he can gain experience and confidence in psychotherapy. The other methods described are quicker and more generally useful, and they can be applied later when one feels competent to make use of them.

The functional case is easily recognisable and when confronted by one during the ordinary surgery hours, it is as well to content oneself with taking a full list of symptoms. If these do not in any way suggest an acute and serious physical lesion, the patient should be put off until more time can be spent on his case. It should be explained that his condition is in no way dangerous, but that he must have a full and complete examination which will take the best part of an hour. An appointment time is given and he is asked to bring with him a specimen of urine. He may be given a drug to tide him over until he is seen again. There is no doubt that sedatives often do help the neurotic, but it is on a par with giving aspirin for toothache. An anodyne is a necessity if no dentist is available ; but there is no doubt as to the proper place of radical treatment. Patients often ask for a tonic. It is as well to point out that there is no cure for nerves to be found in a medicine bottle ; medicine may help, but it does not cure. This can be explained to the patient by using the parable of a fracture. "If you came to me with a broken leg, and I offered you a pair of crutches, you would not be satisfied. If on the other hand I first set the broken bone, you would gratefully accept the crutches too, knowing that they are a temporary measure to tide you over until your leg is better. Any medicine I may give you is a crutch. It may be useful to you, but it is no cure. I don't mind you taking it if you look upon it as a crutch which you will later discard when you can stand on your own feet." If the patient asks questions it may be necessary to evade them by saying he must wait until there is time to discuss things fully. The situation requires tact, as the average neurotic is used to being put off, and hustled out of the surgery. He must be made to feel that his complaints are taken seriously. Once he realises that the doctor is really interested in his case he usually agrees readily to postpone further discussion until the special session.

The First Session or Diagnostic Interview

For the first session at least three quarters of an hour should be allowed. If necessary the list of symptoms should be amplified and the patient should be encouraged to talk. This may seem a dangerous process to those who feel that the neurotics talk too much and wallow in a description of their symptoms. Experience proves that it is important to let the patient get everything off his chest. It gives him satisfaction to be allowed to talk at length and once he has done so he becomes less garrulous. It should be noted that after this he is not encouraged to talk about his feelings: it is the cause of those feelings that is important. In subsequent interviews if a patient starts off describing symptoms he is told they are already known, and so he is guided on to a more profitable subject. When he has exhausted his list of complaints he should be asked about each part he has omitted, so that a full list of his symptoms is obtained. It creates an embarrassing situation if after a negative examination, one has reassured the patient and he then says, "I forgot to tell you about a singing in my left ear. What causes that?"

Having compiled a list of symptoms, a history of the present illness, past complaints, accidents and operations should be taken. I usually record a brief family history round the family tree as it makes for easy reference.

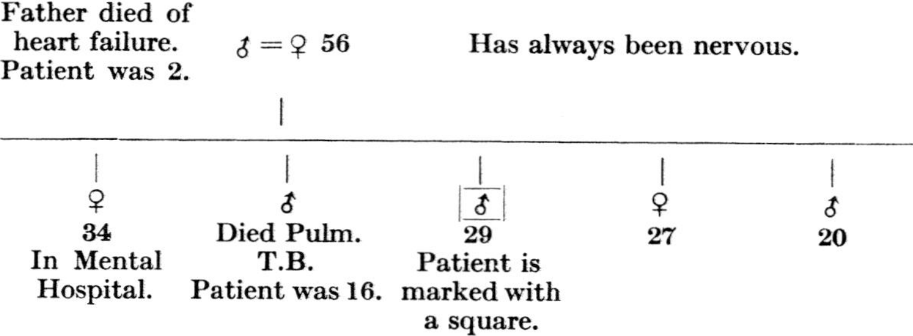

When members of the family have died, the patient's age at the time of bereavement is important, because a family crisis may well have a bearing on the neurosis.

It is useful to ask the patient for his earliest memory. Few can remember much before the age of five. The point of this question will be seen later. He should be asked how he did at school, what class he reached and what examinations were taken and a detailed history of his employment since leaving school should be noted. The man who has worked steadily at one job, or has only changed his work for really adequate reasons is a far better personality type than the rolling stone, and the prognosis is so much the better. Intelligence and the ability to persist at a job of work are points which favour the success of psychotherapy.

His habits such as smoking, drinking and so on, and his interests and hobbies should be noted. Once again the man who has strong interests outside his work, who prefers gardening, sports or collecting butterflies, is better material than the individual who spends all his leisure hours in such passive pursuits as going to the pictures or the local public house. I ask him if he is engaged and what romances he has had. It is unnecessary to ask any embarrassing questions on sex at this stage, as they come so much more easily once the patient has developed confidence : that is, once he has developed a good rapport.*

Then follows a complete physical examination, when special attention can be devoted to any organ which has provoked symptoms. With male patients it is as well to have them completely stripped, so that one can take in the general physique at a glance. The patient's attention should be drawn to any abnormality seen. It may have a bearing on the case, but he is too shy to mention it. One man had a bent penis. When I remarked on this fact he said it had always worried him, and at one time he had toyed with the idea of celibacy as he felt it would be useless. The bent penis in fact played quite a part in his psychological make up. One is not so ruthless with one's female patients who are allowed to retain their knickers. The patient's attitude while being examined is interesting. His attempts to see the sphygmomanometer readings, his remarks as one finishes examining the chest or his optic discs all point to his state of fear, and sometimes reveal fears he has never openly admitted.

If a complete physical examination cannot rule out organic disease and any special investigations have to be made, such as a Wassermann Reaction or an X-ray of the chest, these must be undertaken before psychotherapy can be started.

Once the examination is completed, the patient must be told what has been found. Here it must be stressed that the patient must be told the truth and it must be in words he can understand. If his blood pressure is raised or he has a leaking heart valve, he must be told of these findings and if this condition is not significant, it must be explained to him. "I have examined you thoroughly and I find no abnormality beyond

*Technically this is called a positive transference.

a moderate degree of blood pressure. This has no bearing on your present condition and it really is of no significance. Plenty of people at your age have a raised blood pressure. It may even be the excitement caused by your examination. I am telling you about it because it is my duty to tell you what I find." The truth rarely upsets the patient. There is a popular tradition that doctors always hide signs of real illness from their patients. This is especially supposed to be so if the patient is nervous. Relations often say, "Don't tell him if you do find anything. It will only make him worry". This attitude must be debunked. The patient must be made to realise that his doctor is hiding nothing from him ; and it is not so much disease which worries a patient, but fears of the unknown, which are almost invariably far worse than the disease itself.

In the vast majority of cases the findings are completely negative and the patient can then be told quite simply that he has no bodily disease ; that the symptoms are in fact, not due to disease of any organ but to tension in his mind. The interaction of mind and body is then illustrated by enquiring what happens if he goes to church without a handkerchief, and the correct answer is usually given. It is pointed out that if he can make his nose run by worrying, it is reasonable to suppose that he can, in the same way, upset the rhythm of other organs. A striking example of this may be quoted in a girl who misses a period after being familiar with her boy friend. Once pregnancy has been proved absent, by a negative urine test, the menses soon reappear showing that she had missed her period simply through the fear that she might be pregnant. It can also be pointed out that if we bring our conscious mind to bear on functions like breathing and walking that are normally performed mechanically, we upset the even rhythm. Breathing becomes irregular, one tends to hold one's breath, to sigh or get uneasy feelings in the chest, and all this is readily appreciated by the average patient. He is now in a position to see that nervous tension can produce any number of strange symptoms, pains and sensations and that the next step is to discover the source of the nervous tension in his own mind.

No more than this can be done at the first session but the patient leaves the surgery assured that his problem is really likely to be solved. He has not been treated to such phrases as "There is really nothing wrong with you" or "It's *just* nerves". The first is untrue and the second implies that he is making an undue fuss about a triviality. Another popular fallacy may need attention at this stage. It is commonly believed that a neurosis is rather disgraceful, in that the patient is lacking in will power. Experience in psychiatry shows this to be quite unfair, but the laity and many doctors believe it to be true. The patient should be made to feel that in reporting to a medical man he has taken a wise step and reassured that even if all his symptoms cannot be explained at once their origin will be elucidated at subsequent sessions.

On the other side, at the end of the interview the doctor himself has a rough idea of the material he is dealing with, and how profitable psychotherapy is likely to be. If the patient's past health, scholastic achievements, family history and employment records are good, he is obviously good material and should readily respond to treatment. If his records are bad, he will probably prove a difficult and disappointing subject. In other words some idea has been formed as to the probable prognosis ; and in the light of that, the busy practitioner can decide how much time is worth devoting to the case. If the problem appears difficult, a beginner would be well advised to pass the patient on to a psychiatrist. To gain confidence one should confine one's first efforts in psychotherapy to the best cases. The case history itself, or the patient's behaviour, may have suggested grounds for further probings, and all through one has had ample opportunity to get the feel of the case. Anxiety states, like depression and mania have their own "feel". This is expressed by the patient's obvious interest in the treatment. The diagnostic interview usually starts off with a deluge of symptoms, but once psychotherapy has been started the patient tends to show more interest in that process than in his original complaints. As treatment progresses this becomes more and more obvious. He asks questions not about his symptoms but on topics which are far removed from them. He gets really loquacious as he enlarges on his difficulties at work or in the home, and the pain in his chest seems to be forgotten. He is eager to co-operate and willing to return for treatment whenever necessary. He is keen to assist in piecing together the various pieces of evidence which explain the whole condition.*

A co-operative attitude strongly suggests an anxiety state. The task of the doctor is to prove this by the discovery of a problem which has been wholly or partially buried in the subconscious. Exposure of this problem should give considerable relief to the patient.

The first session described above is straightforward and easy, and need be neither much longer nor more complicated than an insurance examination, provided the end objectives are kept clearly in mind. The subsequent sessions are more difficult for the beginner because the efficiency of one's method depends largely on one's experience. As in most branches of medicine, book knowledge is not enough and a beginner in psychotherapy is like a novice in anæsthetics not knowing quite where his patient is or what to do next. The greatest difficulty is to know how to make the patient talk and if the patient is of the quiet uncommunicative type psychotherapy can be a distinct embarrassment. In early days it is therefore helpful to use a method in which the physician fills in time doing a great deal of talking himself, if necessary. I found that a description of mechanisms often interested the patient at the beginning of the second session after he has had time to meditate upon the vagaries of his running nose and irregular breathing. Turning from the effect of mind on body for a moment, to the mind itself, one can explain how memories appear to be more or less under one's control but that there are memories that appear to have been forgotten. These are

*Psychotherapy is not unlike playing with a jigsaw puzzle. One does not need all the pieces in order to get a good idea of the completed picture.

stored in the deeper part of the mind and are not readily available at will. The earliest memory (obtained at the first session) is usually about 5 years, although a child is very lively and aware long before that age, and very obviously what happens to a child before 5 years has an important influence on his whole life. "Give me a child until he is seven and he will always be a Catholic" was a Jesuit belief, basically true. Memories become submerged and hidden from our direct control but remain a part of our mind content just as the submerged nine-tenths of an iceberg remain part of the whole. At the age of 5 years a child goes to school, and has to absorb a vast amount of knowledge and face innumerable new experiences. This flood of new impressions assists in the repression of infantile memories. The child is looking forward to growing up and reminders of helpless infancy are willingly forgotten.

A short talk along these lines may provoke some discussion or revive the memory of some experience which the patient proceeds to expound. If, however, the patient still shows no response one can embark on a few simple and interesting case histories, illustrating the way in which the resolution of difficulties in other people has led to the clearing of their physical symptoms. This shows the patient that he is in no way peculiar, and that his doctor has successfully treated cases before. There is indeed a real hope of recovery ahead. It also gives the patient some idea of what the doctor is trying to do. Very often at the end of some such case history the patient will say, "When you told me that story I was reminded of something", and forthwith you have your patient talking along the lines you want him to talk. It is important to accept without emotion or criticism any experiences or ideas that the patient may relate, and to make him feel that his reactions and ideas are understandable and indeed, common place. A case such as this can be quoted.

Mrs. J.M. was a young woman of 27 with a baby two months old. I was asked to see her by her husband because he was worried about her as she was run down. Physical examination revealed nothing abnormal. I told her of my negative findings and I explained that when one found no physical cause for symptoms one had to go further and see what was worrying the patient, as worry can cause such things, and explained how memories and worries may be forgotten. Rather reluctantly she admitted she had a worry. When I asked her what it was, she said "You will laugh at me". I told her nothing ever surprised or shocked me, and I never laughed at any idea how bizarre it might appear. Then she told me she had a feeling that she wanted to throw her baby out of the window. That, I told her was a phobia, a very common symptom of nervous illness. The form was unusual but the symptom common place. I assured her it was something I would be able to relieve and I was quite sure she would never actually do such a thing. It was a fear, not a real threat. I made an appointment and she came to see me at the surgery. I talked to her about other cases and showed her the kind of thing that could cause symptoms, and she responded with her life story which was most interesting. She supposed she was the illegitimate daughter of some doctor ; but she was not sure. At 2 she was adopted by a fine type of working class family and tagged on to the end of a family of four children. She had spent her first two years in B., a sizable city. Until she was 14 the name of B. made her feel queer, she did not know why. At 8 she heard her foster-mother talking to someone at the door. Childlike she looked out to see who it was and found a man on the doorstep. In the background was a van from B. She became panic-stricken, ran upstairs and locked herself in her bedroom for 4 hours. At 14 her mother took her aside and told her she was not her own child, but adopted. She astounded her mother by saying that she knew that already. Her mother asked her who had told her, but she said no one, she just knew.

The explanation of these incidents is obvious. Consciously she did not know of her early years, but subconsciously she was well aware of her early years at B. She knew she was different from her foster-brothers and sisters. She had always been fearful of B., because she felt that was where she really belonged and that one day someone would reclaim her. Hence her panic at the age of 8. Her mother's confidence about her adoption, and her reassurance that she had really come to stay, removed from her forever the fear of B. She even dared visit the place, and although it did not attract her, it had ceased to fill her with a morbid fear.*

When she came down for her second session, I asked her if she had had any dreams. She told me she had dreamed she was putting a wreath on the grave of a brother who had died 7 years before. This boy had been killed by falling in a quarry accident. Before I could ask or explain any meaning in the dream, she burst into tears and it was a minute or so before she could compose herself to speak. Tears are usually an indication that one is getting close to the heart of the problem.

She told me the story of her brother's death and how her family had always blamed the foreman in charge. Then she added, that the foreman was her father-in-law as in spite of the ill-feeling between the two families she had married into the "hated" family. I discussed the accident and, as a neutral hearer, I told her I could not see how her father-in-law was to blame. I pointed out how blaming other people helped to ease the family's feelings, just as a child will punish the floor when he has fallen down.

When she came to see me the third time, she said she was quite better. On going home her husband had asked her what we had discussed and she told him all about it. Much to her surprise he wasn't a bit angry, but he had affirmed it was foolish to blame his father. The explanation of the case was that between this excellent couple was the spectre of the dead brother. She had never dared discuss the matter with her husband. Once she had done so, and found he was quite reasonable about it, her anxiety was at an end. "How do you account for the phobia of wanting to throw your baby out of the window?" I asked. "I have an explanation for that too",

---

*Children are more logical than we often imagine. If this child had been told of the adoption earlier, her fears would have been dispelled just as easily.

she told me. "I never realised how much my mother must have suffered until I had a son of my own : and don't forget, my brother died by falling."

This case in all took up less than three hours of my time, and the patient has had no further trouble.

A great deal may be accomplished by this method which can be described as exploratory conversation. The physician, carefully avoiding all moral judgment, watches for clues and in self defence develops a "patter" to fill in awkward silences. Experience soon shows the kind of patter which produces the most helpful response.

Once a practitioner has, by the process of exploratory conversation, built up confidence through the successful treatment of a few of his own cases, he will probably feel able to embark on more organised systems of therapy. These new methods will enable him to circumvent silence and the difficulties innate in an uncommunicative patient, by having different avenues of approach.

These methods are as follows :—

(1) Direct approach. This consists of correlating in time the advent of symptoms with adverse circumstances.

(2) Approach by observing the purpose served by the neurosis.

(3) Approach by observing the emotion expressed by the neurosis. (Organ language).

(4) Approach through dream interpretation.

(5) Approach through free association.

The Direct Approach. This process is started after taking the case history and making a physical examination. The patient is asked when his symptoms first started, and a search is made for psychic trauma which immediately preceded their advent. If he complains of a pain in the chest which started when he was a prisoner of war, he is encouraged to relate some of his experiences during that time, his hopes, his fears, and what he thought was the matter with him then. With adequate probing one can often find the basis for the onset of the neurosis.

Hidden psychic traumata, which could have provoked anxiety, and which were revealed by this method are well illustrated in the following cases.

J.S. was a man of 24 who was suffering from effort syndrome. His first attack came on in Switzerland, where he was awaiting repatriation as an escaped prisoner of war. He remembered that he was then writing to his aunt, but as the letter had been written some eighteen months prior to my interview he had no idea of its contents. I told him that something in his letter had upset him, and that if it was important enough to upset him it could not really have been forgotten. I told him that if we left the subject and talked of other things the memory might return.

"What do you think of your aunt?" I asked him. "I'm very fond of her", was his immediate reply. We discussed the old lady. She was his foster-mother, but, being a maiden lady, she was called aunt. She had been kindness itself to him, but he was anxious to break away and stand on his own feet. After half an hour of discussion I repeated my question, "What do you think of your aunt?" "It's a mixture of gratitude and indifference", was his reply. In his first answer he had given his conscious feelings or the orthodox reply which was expected of him. His real feelings had to be stimulated before they were obvious, especially to himself. We broke off the session at this point, but as he reached the door he remarked, "I know what was in that letter". He told me he was replying to a request from his aunt. She had made him the generous offer of a farm which she wanted him to take over. If he accepted the offer he would lose his independence for which he was striving. It was not easy to word a letter refusing the offer without hurting her feelings and appearing ungrateful. Syncope came as a temporary respite from his struggle. He collapsed in some way and his friends sent for a doctor. In childhood he had had enteric fever with deep femoral thrombosis. The Swiss doctor declared he had had a heart attack due to an embolus. This diagnosis, which was obviously wrong, had fixated the idea of heart disease and effort syndrome had developed. In this case the probing back to the onset of the symptoms was rewarded by the discovery of the real cause of his troubles. Once the whole field of his problems had been discussed, he lost his fear of heart disease, and his attacks ceased. He improved generally as his self-confidence returned.

Mrs. T.G. came to see me complaining of a headache. She was depressed and could not sleep at nights ; her rest being broken by unpleasant dreams. She had difficulty in concentrating and noise, including the wireless, upset her.

At the first therapeutic session, I found she was an intelligent young woman with an excellent work record. She had been married for two years and was living at home. Her husband was in the B.O.A.C. and she only saw him at intervals. She affirmed that the separation did not worry her unduly. No cause for her depression could be found until I noted that the symptoms started soon after an abortive attempt to find a house. They had bought a place in Scotland and just when they planned to move in, her husband was moved to the South of England, and the house had to be re-sold. This incident was discussed at length. She was an uncomplaining woman and had kept things to herself. However with encouragement she admitted that for her, married life was a farce as she saw her husband for only 4 days in every month. She had never complained, either to him or to her own people. I discussed the effect of bottling up one's feelings and I pointed out how her symptoms had in fact coincided with a major disappointment. She was seen again two years later at the ante-natal clinic. She told me then that once her frustrations had been discussed openly she had felt much better. She was looking forward to having a baby and she was soon to join her husband in a more settled existence as he had taken a job with a house attached to it.

Approach Through Observing the Purpose of Neurosis. All neuroses are purposeful, although the motive usually lies at a subconscious level. The injured miner who is on compensation is very liable to prolong his symptoms indefinitely. While he is on compensation he has an easy job which keeps him away from the dangers of the coal face where his accident occurred. Such a motive is usually subconscious and the patient has no insight into his condition. He will say how he longs to be back at his old job, and will complain how much money he is losing by doing light work. Any suggestion that his symptoms were motivated would be met with great indignation and denial, though it does not take a psychiatrist to see the motivation. One miners' leader told me how a man who had just pocketed the cheque for his lump sum compensation said naïvely, "Now I must try and get my old job back".

The purpose behind a neurosis is often clear to the psychotherapist long before the patient is aware of such a mechanism, and the task of the doctor is tactfully to bring him face to face with the real problem. The best course is to guide the patient so that he works it out for himself, but in general practice time will not always allow for this; and once adequate rapport is established and the patient has a grasp of elementary psychology, it is often successful if he is confronted with the problem as the therapist sees it.

Mrs. C.F., aged 30, suffered from severe attacks of palpitations and shaking for which there was no physical cause. One day after several sessions she announced that she had worked it all out.

The attacks started at the age of eight when she was at school. They excluded her from games which she never enjoyed. In later life she had attacks at the cinema. On reflection she realised that these attacks always came on when she was with her mother, and never on the rare occasions when she was allowed to go with her own friends. The attacks which upset her while I was seeing her prevented her from taking back her elder child which her mother had adopted. She was never well enough to have two small children. As soon as she felt better and was prepared to make the effort, another attack would appear and the problem would be evaded once more. This was the patient's own idea of the actual mechanism : and as far as I could see it was correct.

L.B. was a captain in the W.A.A.S.* holding a responsible post. When I was called in to see her as M.O. for the district I diagnosed her condition as influenza. Her commanding officer asked to see me and told me she was very worried about the girl. She had always been a model of efficiency, but over the past few weeks there had been a marked falling off in her capacity for work. It was suggested that she had been overworking and needed a holiday. Armed with this information I spent my next visit taking a history of the case, and I started on a psychological approach. Her illness dated from the receipt of a letter from her mother asking her to get transferred to her home town, to be near her, as all the rest of the family had left home. Her attitude to her mother was one of antagonism. At school she had ambitions of getting in the hockey team, but mother would not allow her to play. At 20 she had taken a young man home, and her mother was very rude to him. The girl sided with the boy, left home and married him. Marriage was a failure and she blamed her mother for this. If only she had given them more time to court, instead of precipitating a rushed marriage, things would have been different. Now she had a good responsible post which she thoroughly enjoyed and mother was "plucking at her heart strings" and calling her home. This state of indecision had lowered her efficiency at work and in the end made her ill. The purpose of the neurosis was to cast a smoke screen over the whole problem and to delay a difficult decision. Discussion made her appreciate the situation as a whole. She decided to carry on with her work and wrote to tell her mother that she could not leave her work which was of national importance. Her efficiency recovered without any sick leave.

Approach by Observing what Emotion is Expressed by a neurosis. To a beginner in psychiatry it seems far fetched to talk about "organ language". In actual fact our organs can some-

*Equivalent to the A.T.S. in South Africa.

times express our real feelings very adequately. One woman was devastated to hear that her husband in the forces had decided to leave her. She never actually cried about it but she developed a weeping eczema of her hands. Her hands wept for her. Effort syndrome can portray a broken heart. A commando who found it difficult to settle down into the hum-drum office job developed asthma, to show how constricted life had become for him. Women who have a dread of pregnancy often complain of vertigo—a fear of falling. There are two ways in which a woman can fall and the symptom is very expressive.

The following case illustrates the method of approach.

S.A. was a young soldier of 26 who was referred to me for persistent vomiting. No physical cause for his complaint could be found. He had escaped from a P.O.W. cage in Italy and for a year had lived the life of a bandit. The day after he had reached the British lines—and safety, he started vomiting. I could find no reason at first, so I flung out at him, "What does vomiting express?" He could not see my point, so I told him it could be a sign of disgust. I related the story of an Englishman who, having enjoyed a French dish of frogs' legs, was sick when he was told what he had eaten. My patient opened up at once. Talking of disgust, he said he had never been so shocked in his life as when he was rescued. The Fascist mayor of an Italian village had entertained him with the object of trying to make a good impression. When my patient heard English voices outside he went out and greeted a tank commander. They smoked a cigarette and arranged a rendezvous, as the tank had to complete a patrol before picking him up. When the tank moved on he returned to the house to find the mayor and his wife and family had all been butchered by patriots. Their brains bespattered the walls and their bellies were ripped up. He said he had never seen such a disgusting sight in his life. The next day he started vomiting.

The correlation of symptoms and circumstances was very instructive in this case. He had been a bilious child, and with some hesitation he produced this story. His father had died when he was 5. His mother took to drink, but he didn't realise this until he was about 7. He found her sitting at the table so ataxic that she could not hit her mouth with her spoon as she ate. He told me he would never forget the feeling of dismay and disgust that swept over him. So far as he could recollect his bilious bouts came on after this incident, and it looked as if they served a very useful purpose in forcing his mother's attention on him from time to time. Later, as a clerk in an insurance firm, he frequently lost work owing to his attacks. He did not like the work, and he felt that his talents were being exploited and when the director of his firm visited his office he sought an interview with him. He evidently made a good impression, as he became the private secretary to this man, his salary was raised, and he had no more attacks of vomiting. He had never correlated his symptoms with his environment. The comparison showed how vomiting on each occasion had expressed disgust.

While on week-end leave this man had an unpleasant experience. He was to visit an uncle, but when he got there he found his host had committed suicide and the family were in a turmoil. I asked him if he had been sick. "I felt nauseated", he said, "but after our talks I felt I should be able to control myself, and I never actually vomited."

Dream Interpretation. It is not possible in a book of this nature to give more than the merest outline on this subject. My object is to describe a few basic principles which will allow the general practitioner who is interested to make use of dreams in psychotherapy. Dreams are sometimes a useful short cut in treatment, and Freud described them as the highway to the subconscious. Dreams are in fact messages from the subconscious mind ; usually heavily disguised so that the subject is unaware of the real meaning.

The actual dream story is the manifest content of the dream. The meaning hidden behind the dream is known as the latent content. All dreams have a meaning ; but it may not be readily apparent or there may be more than one explanation.

Most dreams express some desire and they are in fact a wish fulfilment. The P.O.W. living on potato soup dreams of Christmas dinner at home. The thirsty man in a desert dreams of babbling brooks and so on.

The wish expressed in these dreams is obvious, but in others it may be lightly or heavily disguised. A married woman living on a lonely farm used frequently to dream she was back in the office. When asked the advantages of office life, she described them as freedom and a social life, the very things she was denied in her married life.

H.W. was a man with effort syndrome and when asked if he had any dreams to report, he replied he had a short one but it had no meaning. I asked him for it and he said he was just watering a tree. When I asked him what kind of a tree it was, he replied it was some flowers under the tree. They were violets. I asked him the name of his girl friend and it was Iris ; the same colour as the violets. Iris had married another man and was regretting that step. She was still in love with my patient and he was in love with her. Thus in the manifest of the dream he is watering violets : but the latent meaning is he wishes he could cultivate and care for Iris. No doubt Freudians would go a step further in analysis and suggest that he watered or micturated on the violets to express his desire to copulate with Iris.

More than one meaning can be woven into a dream, and if patients produce dreams which shock them, one must be prepared to reassure them. They may be shocked by the manifest, but the latent content is usually quite harmless.

A soldier dreamed he climbed a tower and in the top room found his sister lying in bed. He had intercourse with her and on waking was filled with remorse over the dream as he felt it was shameful. The sister in the dream had died in childbirth 10 years before. His wife was pregnant. So the dream actually expressed a desire and a fear : a desire to be with his wife and a fear lest she should suffer in childbirth like his sister.

Dreams of dead persons after death are usually the wish fulfilment, the desire to have them back again. Dreams of living people being dead usually express a death wish for that person.

If a girl dreams that her mother has died, it may well express the wish that her mother could be removed, leaving father to his daughter.* If however a mother dreams that her child dies or is injured it may not be a death wish but a warning. The voice of conscience often speaks to us in our dreams, and such a dream might well indicate as follows: "Check up on your attitude to, and care for, your child, or this may happen. Are you paying sufficient attention to the child?" This warning or reminder type of dream is not uncommon. A patient dreamed the telephone was ringing. When he picked up the receiver, all he could hear was a woman at the other end sobbing. He recognised the woman as his sister. On waking he realised that he had had four letters from her awaiting an answer. The dream reminded him and warned him, "If you don't answer your sister she will be upset".

During psychotherapy the mind is stirred up and memories which have sunk deep down start floating into the higher reaches and may emerge in the form of dreams. It is with this in mind that I ask some of my patients to write down any dreams they may have between sessions, as useful information may emerge during sleep.

Mrs. M.O., a woman of 37, came to see me about a phobia which had troubled her since she was 13. We could find no trigger incident to put the neurosis in motion at that age. I told her I was confident that we would find something, and I asked her to remember her dreams. The next session she came back and said she had dreamed someone had left a brown-paper parcel on the doorstep. She awoke and found herself in an awful state. "I know now what upset me at 13", she said. Then she proceeded to describe how one day when she

*See previous Chapter.

came home from school she had found a brown-paper parcel on the kitchen table. She was curious and looked inside. It contained soiled linen and a placenta. She did not know what it was, but she felt guilty about the whole affair and associated it correctly with the birth of her youngest brother. Soon afterwards her periods started and the same feelings of guilt assailed her in spite of her mother's meagre assurance that it was a normal event. When I questioned her about these memories she affirmed that, as far as she could remember, she had never given the matter thought since her marriage seven years previously.

A dream may depict a situation in the form of a cartoon. A girl in doubt as to which lover to accept may dream of choosing between two cars. A man who had been in the regular army for many years was to be discharged on health grounds. He was an N.C.O. but had never undertaken much responsibility ; and he didn't relish the idea of standing on his own feet in "civvy street". He dreamed he was travelling in a car with his father, and he was enjoying the ride through lovely country. Suddenly he found himself driving the car down a steep and dangerous hill on his own and he awakened in terror. Father stood for the army, and as long as father was with him, or he with father, all was well. On his own he was full of misgivings.

A woman of 37 was in a severe anxiety state which had lasted for some 3 years. There were two possible causes of this condition. Soon after her husband returned from the army she developed a vaginal discharge. Her husband also had a discharge and they both suspected venereal disease. After investigation these fears were allayed but the patient was very shaken by the experience. Then she quarrelled violently with her next door neighbours, a couple who had always treated her like a daughter. They slandered her on every possible occasion and were making her life a misery. The whole picture was well portrayed in a dream. The neighbour walked into my patient's garden to show someone the local cemetery at the bottom of the lawn. A cemetery mysteriously appeared in the dream. The neighbour then returned on his own, spoke to my patient and started passing water in front of her, on her lawn. She was angry and called her husband, who attacked the neighbour and knocked him out. The husband was worried in case he had killed him, but my patient knew that he was just shamming.

This dream summed up the situation. There was a grave-yard of memories round their house. The neighbour's contemptuous attitude and lack of manners was clearly cartooned in what happened.

No essay on dreams would be complete without some mention of symbolism. Freud contended that symbols were an international language in dreams. The phallus was represented by a knife, a horn, a stick or a tower. The female counterpart was represented by a room or some receptacle. Sexual desire was shown up in scenes of flying or swimming or climbing stairs and so on. It is not appropriate to deal fully with this matter here. Further information on the subject should be sought in Freud's own works or works by his followers. But no one can make a study of dream material without being impressed by the occurrence of such symbols.

I had a patient who had had two severe acute schizophrenic episodes. His hallucinations were startling and terrifying. During one of these attacks he was called upon by the Almighty (by his Christian name) to sever off his penis. He obeyed the order with a razor blade in his bath and felt fine as soon as it was over. When I saw him he was perfectly rational and normal except for the missing organ. He told me he had repeatedly had dreams of being on a ship all alone. Suddenly snakes would appear and he would have to scramble up the mast for safety. The loathsome creatures followed him and he would awake screaming with terror. This dream had afflicted him periodically as long as he could remember. One day he came in triumphant, he had had the snake dream again ; the first since his "operation".* This time he found

*When this patient was admitted to hospital after the loss of his penis, a surgeon who examined him remarked "But you cut off the wrong thing". That

himself armed with a sword and he was severing the creatures right and left, quite a delightful sensation, he assured me.

Another man who was a kind of Don Juan, told me of a dream he had had. He was taking his latest girl friend for a walk and they came to a weird city of towers. He realised he owned a tower in this city and they set out to look for it. It was bigger and better than all the rest and he asked his girl to admire it.

"How did you recognise it as your own ?" I asked him.

"By the big shiny red dome on top" was his naïve reply.

Alcoholism is often an expression of a latent homo-sexual tendency. In the army I was confronted by a boy with a bad alcoholic history and an inexplicable pain in his rectum. The first dream he produced for me was as follows :—

"I was running away from a military policeman when I came to a flight of steps. I ran up the steps and at the top was a door. A kind faced woman pulled me inside and I found a party going on. The woman's daughter was to be married. She asked me to dance with the bride but I refused and said I would rather have a glass of brandy." This dream vividly portrayed his make up in symbols. He was chased by that male of males the policeman—the father substitute. Sexual desire was expressed by going upstairs. When he was offered a young girl he refused her, and asked for a drink instead. The diagnosis of a sexual neurosis with ano-neurotic symptoms was clearly portrayed by the dream. These dreams convinced me more than anything else that there are symbols in dreams which can be very useful in dream interpretation, but in general practice one cannot use deep therapy and rarely descends to the Freudian depths, so that symbols, although useful to the therapist, are rarely explained to patients, but the wish fulfilment dream or the situation

---

night the patient tried to castrate himself but it was too painful even for him. Such jocularity over a very serious issue was obviously quite out of place. This incident emphasises the need for all branches of the profession to have some psychiatric sense and appreciation.

dream, are fully explained.   In other words only the simplest forms of dream analysis are practicable as far as the general practitioner is concerned.

Free Association. This is not a method that I use frequently with my patients, but it is useful when one comes up against resistance. In brief, the patient is taught to relax and to allow ideas to flow through his mind without any attempt at conscious memory or synthesis. I do not like to have to use this method as it is time consuming and only applicable to long term cases which are a great burden in general practice. I usually, however, keep an odd one on my books because an occasional cure in an apparently hopeless case is very satisfying. One patient was a woman with severe vaginismus of ten years' duration. A gynæcologist had advised a plastic operation which I felt was a hopeless procedure so I persevered with psychotherapy and was eventually rewarded. Pregnancy occurred, the labour was an easy one, and now the patient's sexual life is normal after more than 10 years of married virginity.

The patient is made to lie on a couch and is taught how to relax his body. First one arm is relaxed beginning at the fingers and working up through the wrist and the elbow to the shoulder. The other arm is then tackled, then the legs, the belly, chest muscles and the face and the patient is told to close his eyes as if he is asleep. Before instructing a patient it is as well to try it out oneself. I asked a physiotherapist to put me into a state of relaxation and I copy her methods. It requires practice on the part of both doctor and patient. I find that successful relaxation is not easily achieved but that after three of four sessions the patient can co-operate fully and even if complete relaxation is absent useful work can be done.

J.H., a man of 37, complained of queer feelings in his head and vertigo which kept him off work. He was loath to accept a psychiatric diagnosis, but I persisted with therapy and he improved. One day he arrived in a great state of agitation and very angry. He had had an attack in one of the local public houses which made nonsense of all my suggestions. He was with his friends and his domestic troubles, the cause of his neurosis, were completely out of his mind. He was angry and resistant and no progress could be made.

I tried free association. As he lay somewhat relaxed on the couch, I made him go over in detail what happened to him in the public house. He told me what he had drunk, what he had talked about and whom he had met. L.A. was there. He had the same job as the patient, and the same domestic problem—an unfaithful wife. He saw the connection, and when I next saw him he was much better and more amenable to treatment. Free association had helped where discussion across the desk would have meant a deadlock.

In the army I was confronted by a young airman aged 24. He had attacks of emotionalism which were quite beyond his control and without any apparent provocation he would burst into tears. He was of German descent and his parents were against his joining up as their sympathies were with the Nazis. He waited until he was 21 and then joined the South African Air force. He was an air gunner and had about 20 sorties to his credit before the war ended. While awaiting to return to South Africa, he was working on the airfield clearing up rubbish when a live round which had been thrown by accident on to the burning litter, exploded and gave him a flesh wound in the thigh. He was sent to hospital and repatriated to South Africa. While in hospital his attacks started and he dare not go back to his parents while they lasted.

Routine history taking produced no clear cause for his attacks so I resorted to free association. On the second session of free association, when he was well relaxed, I told him he was back in the Italian hospital. He had told me in detail how he had shared a room with an English soldier who was also a farmer in civil life. I knew the background fairly well. "You are back in the hospital talking to your English comrade ; tell me what is on your mind."

He recited how 'they discussed farming and the different

methods of farming in England and South Africa. He told me he felt homesick and so on. Suddenly he stopped talking. "What are you thinking of now ?" I asked. "I saw a flash of light," he replied. The room was in darkness as they lay in bed and the blackout curtains were drawn back. Someone had fired off a verey light outside. I could see him tensing up on the couch so I felt I was on a good trail. "What does the flash of light remind you of?" I asked. "An aircraft exploding", he replied. "Which aircraft?" I enquired ; and then he told me the following story.

Just before the war ended his plane was loaded up and they were due for a sortie. An hour before the flight began he was taken off his plane and a substitute gunner was put in his place. He discussed the trip with this man, and later from the air strip he saw the plane start off. It taxied across the drome but something went wrong. It crashed, burst into flames and then a few minutes later the bomb load blew up. Then he divulged that as a gunner he was responsible for retracting the forward single wheel. In his plane there was a knack in doing this and he had failed to tell his substitute. In his own mind this memory lapse had caused the disaster and all his friends had been killed. His conscience was loaded with guilt which he had tried hard to repress and the guilt had emerged as attacks of crying. He felt much better after he had revealed this to me but his attacks did not cease altogether. On one occasion I witnessed one, while on a ward round. His lips started quivering and his eyes filled with tears. I took him into a side ward and made him lie down on a bed and relax and his emotionalism soon left him. One must be tensed up to produce emotion in any form. One tenses before anger. It is impossible to be angry when one relaxes. In the same way, I argued, this tearful emotion would respond to proper relaxation—a trick he had learned during free association. A week later he asked if he might see me. He was very pleased with himself as he told me he had mastered his attacks at last. He had been in the town lunching with friends. He had just left them when he felt an attack coming on. He decided he must do something so he dived into a milk bar and started eating ice cream. While he was eating he thought back deliberately over the conversation he had had with his friends at lunch. They had talked of atom bombs. He analysed the whole situation and he decided he hated flying and was scared to death of it. He had never dared to admit this even to himself before. Once he had made this admission, he felt better in himself and no attack emerged. A feeling of confidence came over him, so much that he took it upon himself to come and tell me all about it. He was confident he had mastered his attacks because he himself had worked out an explanation for them. The war was over, and there was no need to fly again in any case.

In this patient free association revealed a guilt situation which had been repressed. The airman was encouraged to face up to a "skeleton" which he had kept hidden away. This encouraged him to do further auto-analysis which resulted in a return of self confidence and an amelioration of the symptoms. At his own request he left to go back to his parents, shortly afterwards.

Hypnosis and narco-analysis are other means which can be used to circumvent a resistance ; but I feel they are beyond the scope of a general practitioner whose time is so seriously limited. If, after using all the methods described, a deadlock is reached in a patient who ought to improve, the situation should be reviewed. Is the condition really an anxiety state, or is the patient for some reason inaccessible to psychotherapy ? The diagnosis must be sought among the following conditions, which will be dealt with in subsequent chapters.

Cases which are Not Anxiety States.
   (1) Endogenous depression (common).
   (2) Schizophrenia (rare).

Cases in which the Patient is Inaccessible to Psychotherapy.
   (1)   The neurosis is too profitable to be abandoned, *i.e.*
         Compensation neurosis.
         Primary hypochondriasis.

(2) The patient lacks insight, *i.e.* psychopathic states, especially hysteria.

(3) The patient's intelligence is inadequate for psycho-therapy, *i.e.* mental defect.

If the practitioner feels he has reached an impasse, he should refer the case on to a psychiatrist, where his case history and his impressions will be most valuable and time saving for the specialist. If the case is a treatable type of anxiety state, the consultant may be able to suggest lines of approach ; but if the case is beyond the scope of a general practitioner the patient will be taken off his hands and treated elsewhere.

REFERENCE

(i) Roland Dalbiez. Psychoanalytic Method and Doctrine of Freud.

CHAPTER IV

NEUROTIC SYNDROMES

BEFORE leaving the subject of anxiety states a few more typical examples are worthy of consideration. As a student one was taught that pain, fever, and vomiting were very suggestive of an acute appendicitis. These symptoms and signs form a clear cut clinical picture. A few neuroses have a clear cut symptomatology and psychopathology, and, because of their typical form, I have called them neurotic syndromes. Once one has resolved such a neurosis, the same approach and method can readily be used on a similar case.

Phobia of Venereal Disease

In my experience, this is one of the easiest and the most gratifying neuroses to treat. I propose describing it in some detail, because to anyone starting out on psychotherapy, the treatment is straightforward and the result usually most satisfactory. The tyro in psychotherapy needs to try his art on cases which have a good prognosis. The satisfactory recovery of a patient rapidly enhances the confidence of the therapist in himself.

The clinical picture is usually that of a man who fastens a peculiarly intense type of worry on to some trivial symptom. For instance, a busy man will wait for several hours in the surgery for an opinion on a minute pimple, or he may seek a second opinion on some trifle or even on a condition which is already clearing. The reason for this is that the patient with venereal disease phobia is constantly on the lookout for some flamboyant revelation of the cause of his secret fears and convictions, and all the time he is harassed by a guilty conscience. The treatment is simply to uncover the worry, and to reduce its intensity. Confession besides being good for the soul, is efficacious for a painfully distracted mind.

In the first place the fear must be exposed as the neurotic with such a phobia rarely states his worry. It has to be suspected and then brought into the open. Next the real disease must be excluded by a thorough examination and the usual clinical tests. Often these cases have already had every conceivable examination performed, and then the ritual of smears and prostatic massage can be omitted, but a Kahn, which is easy to do, helps to reassure the patient and can do no harm. All neurotics are impressed by "a good examination", and reassurance after such always carries more weight than argument and discussion by itself.

Once venereal disease has been excluded it can be explained to the patient that all the symptoms can be accounted for in terms of worry. The nose is not the only organ that runs if one's mind is focused on it. This same process is aggravated by a ritual squeezing of the penis whenever it is seen, in an effort to see if the dreaded discharge is still present. The discharge, which is watery and not frankly purulent, and symptoms such as burning on micturition, a sense of urgency and so on—all these things can be explained in terms of anxiety. The patient is indeed suffering from a conscience reaction. It is suggested to the patient that in his sexual indiscretion, besides acquiring a fear of venereal disease, he hurt his conscience and was ashamed of himself. This shame was intensified by the fear of being found out, once venereal disease became evident. One can go on to explain that we are all made that way. Most people break the law quite freely as long as they know they are safe, but they become very distressed if they feel they have been caught out and that retribution is on the way.

To illustrate and explain the conscience reaction, it is useful to compare this with an orderly room in the army. The culprit is brought before his officer for trial. No matter what the verdict, as he leaves the orderly room he is getting rid of emotional tension. He may be laughing and calling the colonel an old fool, or he may be swearing and declaring himself the victim of the sergeant major's whim. In either case he is getting rid of emotional tension. Either he got off lightly and is pleased, or he is being punished unfairly as it was someone else's fault. Now in the court of conscience, one is the prisoner in the dock and the judge at one and the same time. There are no other actors, no one else on whom we can throw the blame. If one blames the judge one is censuring oneself. Indeed a vicious circle of depression sets in. The harder one is on oneself, the more depressed one gets ; and the more depressed one feels the more one blames oneself. So it must be suggested to the patient he must be more lenient with himself. He is asked if he would give up his best friend because the latter confided in him that he had contracted venereal disease, and the patient invariably states he would never do such a thing. It can then be pointed out that his attitude to himself is really rather prudish or else illogical; he can accept and befriend a comrade who has venereal disease, but he cannot accept himself in that position. The inference is that he is better than his friend, and few people are so superior as to believe that.

While I never suggest that sexual indiscretion is advisable, I point out it is a very understandable mistake. Any decent man should feel towards such matters, "There, but for the Grace of God, go I". If the patient is religious, one can point out that Christ himself was most generous and forgiving towards sins of the flesh. Indeed the story of the woman taken in adultery is one of the most admirable pictures of Jesus in the Bible, and it is sometimes worth repeating.

The object of all this talk is to convince the patient that his conscience has been so upset and injured that he is in actual fact unwilling to forgive himself. The process of explanation seems to give immense relief to the patient and usually before he leaves the surgery he will say, "I feel better already, better than I have felt for weeks".

J.P., a man of 35, came to see me with sychosis barbæ. The rash cleared well on penicillin injections but he was still obviously distressed and asked to see a specialist. He attended the hospital out-patient department but he was disgusted at the offhand way in which he was treated. No blame was really attached to the consultant as by now his rash had cleared. I tried to reassure him but he was still very worried about himself. In the end I told him bluntly, "You behave like a man who is fearful of venereal disease". He protested violently against this suggestion, became agitated and finally burst into tears. Then after binding me to oaths of secrecy, he told me this story. During the war he was in the army and had had to leave his wife and small son behind. While on leave he suspected that his wife had been unfaithful to him as she was so cold towards him. He was compelled to have it out with her and she confessed she was in love with another man. He pleaded with her, and her mother, who knew what was happening ; but it all seemed hopeless and he was threatened with a break up of his marriage. After one particularly distressing leave, in desperation he followed his wife's example and took a lover of his own. He did not enjoy the experience, and was very worried in case he had contracted venereal disease. He had reported sick to one medical officer after another, and had had all the appropriate tests performed but he still refused to be satisfied. Now he was sure the sychosis barbæ was "the disease coming out". I examined him thoroughly and took a Kahn which was negative. I then talked to him along the lines already suggested, and he was rapidly reassured. I have seen him once or twice since with a recrudescence of his skin rash, but he is no longer really worried about it.

J.L., aged 33, came to see me complaining of a pain in his back and general weakness. He had always been a very strong chap, but for a year or so he had gone off. No evidence of physical disease was found, so I questioned him further about when the pain started.

Reluctantly he told me he had overstrained himself with a German girl. He had never had any sexual relations until he was stationed near Hamburg in the R.A.F. Regiment. There it was the custom to have a girl friend, and along with his companions he found a mistress. On the night of his third intercourse with her he "felt something go and his virility left him". He felt he had strained himself and reported to his medical officer. No evidence of venereal disease was found but he continued to feel weak and ill. He never saw the German girl again and he was relieved when he was transferred elsewhere. He reported to medical officers at intervals but no one took his complaint seriously. Some openly laughed at him—but he could not laugh at himself. He came back to England and his back pains grew worse and fibrositis was diagnosed.

A physical examination revealed nothing abnormal. Prostatic smears contained many pus cells but no intracellular organisms. In view of the negative history of discharge it was decided not to pursue tests of gonococci as such would cast doubt on my reassurance. His Wassermann reaction was negative. He felt better after one session of psychotherapy and when questioned about his trouble three years later he told me: "If I had ever needed to attend the surgery I would have come back and seen you, but I have never been ill since then and my back has ceased to worry me".

W.W., a man of 37, was being attended by me for herpes zoster. On my last visit to his house, he asked me rather anxiously to have a look at his lip. As I could see nothing abnormal and as I was in the midst of my round, I told him to rub it with vaseline and come to see me at the surgery, following the principle that when a patient complains a great deal about something which is normal, it usually indicates trouble in his mind of either a neurotic or psychotic nature.

When I saw him at the surgery, he told me he wanted some advice. He had picked up a discharge in the army, and although several doctors had told him he had no infection, he could not be satisfied. He was told the usual story of a conscience reaction and at the end of the session he claimed to feel more satisfied than he had felt for months.

Before closing this section on the phobia of venereal disease, it must be emphasised that in some cases such a phobia may be an expression of endogenous depression, and then the lay out of psychotherapy described above will be quite useless. Indeed the patient's condition may become much worse if the therapist persists in trying to probe into his mind, as the following case shows.

C.E., a soldier aged 34, was obsessed with the idea that he had gonorrhœa. For a year while employed in the Middle East he had seen every available urologist and venereologist. Twice he had submitted to cystoscopy. Before returning home he reported to yet another camp medical officer, who warned him that if he didn't "pull himself together he would end up in the hands of a psychiatrist"! In spite of this warning he ultimately found his way to a neuro psychiatric centre, and he was given psychotherapy. He became worse and developed a great dislike of the therapist and was handed on to me. Because of his attitude and resistance to psychotherapy I came to the conclusion he had an endogenous depression, and after he had had six electro-convulsive treatments, he rapidly returned to normal. When seen seven months later he was back at work and apparently fully recovered.

The patient with anxiety state type of phobia presents with various symptoms which he puts down to venereal disease. He tells one the symptoms but he rarely discloses his real fears. They have to be uncovered and exposed by the therapist. One with depressive phobia, however, usually comes complaining that he has venereal disease, and no negative findings will convince him otherwise. This point bears out Ross's dictum (i) that if a patient talks of sex in the first five minutes of an interview, he is usually psychotic.

Effort Syndrome

This is a condition of cardiac neurosis. The patient complains of a pain in his chest, or palpitations or shortness of breath, or all these symptoms together and many more. He usually readily admits he is worried about his heart. Heart consciousness itself produces many symptoms. The victim notes with increasing apprehension that he gets short of breath on going upstairs. He hears or feels his heart beating at night and dare not sleep in any position which accentuates the pulsations. He palpates his own pulse at intervals and an odd missed beat fills him with fear. All this lies at a conscious level. Deeper down he has a fear of dying, and therefore has a deep seated dread of going unconscious. The thought of an anæsthetic appals him and subconsciously he fears dropping off to sleep, a process psychologically akin to dying. Fainting to the lay mind is pathognomonic of a bad heart ; and in effort syndrome it confirms the patient's fear of cardiac disease. Thus the victim of effort syndrome often has difficulty in dropping off to sleep, not only because his ritual postures are often uncomfortable but also his mind is reluctant to give way to sleep. Frequently just as he is dropping off to sleep he awakes with a convulsive jerk. This frightens him and fear makes his heart pound, so that sleep eludes him more than ever. The patient tends to be more and more careful with himself. Exertion in all forms is evaded and excitement, such as the cinema, is avoided. He becomes flabby physically and empty mentally and so a vicious circle is formed. The less he does the worse he feels, and the worse he feels the more he cuts down on normal activity. The symptoms are vastly different from true organic heart disease.

H.W. was a man of 27. He told me as soon as he came into my consulting room that he had already seen seven doctors. "They all tell me there is nothing the matter with my heart, but I just cannot believe them. I feel I may drop down dead at any moment." I made a physical examination which included an exercise tolerance test. Like my predecessors I found no evidence of organic heart disease. I reassured him about his heart, but pointed out that heart feelings could be produced by means other than actual disease ; and I proceeded to explore his life history more closely. This man had had a cellulitis of his arm, and as a result he had been in and out of hospital for the best part of a year. He had undergone many operations, but took them all as a matter of course until he developed his heart fear. Once that had started, he dreaded anæsthetics. He had only had to have one while in that state of mind and as he recovered consciousness, he told me, his worry was mainly to discover whether he was in heaven or hell as he was quite sure he was dead.

By equating symptoms with environment one could see that his illness developed soon after his girl friend had married a rival. He was so distressed that when he was discharged from hospital following his cellulitis, he joined up and left his home town. In the army he remained well except on one occasion when his unit was bombed. When he came home on leave, all his symptoms returned. He had spoken to his late fiancée and she had told him she still loved him and realised only too late she had made a mistake. Half in fun I told him, "She has broken your heart". It was obvious that the symptoms were activated by a broken romance.

Neither of his parents had died of heart failure, so I asked him if he had ever seen anyone have a heart attack. "Oh yes", he replied. "A fellow once fell off a stool in a pub. I was sitting beside him. He was dead when they picked him up and it was his heart." This incident took place a few weeks before his romance was broken up. It gave him a fright and sensitised him to heart disease. The broken romance precipitated the neurosis which became centred around his own heart.

After two or three sessions of psychotherapy he felt much better. He decided to go and live a long way from his girl friend until they had made up their minds what to do.

Mrs. A.M., a woman aged 42, had called me in because her only child, aged 4, had developed mannerisms and was unduly afraid of cows. I asked her mother to come and see me at the surgery, and it was soon obvious that she herself had a quite severe anxiety state. She complained of pains in her chest and shortness of breath. She had given up cycling and had cut down all her activities. She was convinced it was only a matter of time before she dropped dead. So sure was she of this that she always carried her identity card so that her body would be recognised. She even hid a farewell letter to her husband telling him how to carry on. Such precautions are a measure of how bad she felt. To summarise the case, which in all took four sessions, she was markedly fixated to her father, who had died two years previously from heart disease. As is often the case in neuroses, his illness served as a pattern for her symptoms. So great was her fixation that she was courted for nine years before she would consent to marry at 36. Attracted by her father, she was strongly antagonistic to her invalid mother, who lived at the other side of the town. She visited her mother thrice weekly, but it was an irksome duty and gave her no pleasure. Consciously she strove to be dutiful; subconsciously she hated her mother and resented the attention she had to pay her. This is roughly what must have happened. When she felt tired one day she decided she was not fit enough to make the journey. "I would go if I felt better", was her feeling, and so she stayed at home. The purpose of the neurosis is clear. She gave up cycling, and if she had to use a taxi the visits would be cut down to once a month. As T. A. Ross (i) put it, a neurosis is always a bad bargain in the end. Her feelings excused her certain duties towards her mother, but in the end they made life almost unbearable for the patient herself. Once all this conflict had been clarified at a conscious level the patient felt much better. After the third session she announced herself as well; she could run upstairs and swill the yard in a way she had not done for months. All her fears had left her, and, what is more, her little girl had recovered too.

Unlike venereal disease phobia, effort syndrome has a variable psychopathology, but the symptomatology is similar in most cases. It responds well to psychotherapy, but one cannot expect such a rapid improvement as in previous syndromes.

Nocturnal Eneuresis

No doctor can work long in a general practice without being confronted with this problem. In the vast majority of cases there is a large psychological factor, but unfortunately, unlike venereal disease phobia, it does not respond to any set formula of treatment. An approach which will relieve one patient will fail in another. The reason for the resistance of this common complaint to treatment lies in its complicated origin. Largely psychological it can also have an organic or a physiological basis. Urinary infections, nephritis, and diabetes mellitus are organic factors. Strän Olsen (ii) recently pointed out that hypersomnia can be a cause of eneuresis. The victim is so deeply asleep that the ordinary reflex cell is insufficient to awaken him. However in most cases there is a psychological factor. The patient has failed to throw off an infantile habit at the appropriate age. In my experience the displaced child is more likely to be affected than the youngest sibling. Often one finds the baby immune, whilst the older child or children are the bed wetters. The displaced child looks backwards with longing towards infancy instead of forward to maturity, and the habit is displayed as a token of that longing. This type is fairly obvious at the outset if eneuresis is set in soon after the arrival of a new baby. It is surprising how strong the latent jealousy can be, and to what age it can affect people. One boy of twelve started wetting the bed when his baby sister was three. I discussed the family layout with his mother. The father looked upon the small girl as his special pride and ignored his son, who was severely disciplined. I suggested it might be a longing for the affection and privileges of infancy, and that if she could impress upon him the importance of growing up it might counteract the infantile desires. She acted on my advice by buying him a pair of long trousers and allowing him to stay out until 10.0 p.m. on Scouts nights, and his habit cleared.

I was visiting a house and the mother asked me to see J., a little girl of 5, who was a bed wetter. Her small brother, age 3, was a model of virtue. I explained the latent jealousy motive to the mother and told her to give the child a calendar to mark every dry night. I suggested that when she succeeded in producing seven consecutive crosses she would have some reward. This consultation, made on a round, was of necessity brief, but it was crowned with success. J. won her prize the first week and never thereafter relapsed.

Unfortunately this method, and all the ritual of cutting out drinking after tea, wakening the child at night and so on works in one case with dramatic effect, but is a complete failure in the next two or three.

In some ways adults are easier to treat than children as one can work directly with the patient. With children one talks to the mother who performs the psychotherapy as it were second hand. In adults one can sometimes see a motive which one might not suspect in a child, the motive of revenge. One woman I treated displayed this reaction by wetting the bed when she felt angry with her husband. During psychotherapy I discovered that the man was a keen guinea pig breeder, and his wife felt he spent too much time with them. She remarked on one occasion that she thought he cared more for his guinea pigs than he did for her. She kept a calendar, and some interesting points came to light. She never wet the bed after sexual intercourse, but frequently if her husband was out late with these guinea pigs, or if he had spent all day at a show. If they had any argument and she went to bed upset it always happened. Thus a display of affection on the husband's part prevented eneuresis : but the suggestion of neglect precipitated the reaction. A discussion of the whole situation both with the husband and wife went far to relieve it though it did not produce a complete cure.

My feeling is that the problem is well worth tackling with psychotherapy though there is no clear cut formula. In some cases the discovery of a hidden cause or motive will bring immediate and gratifying results, in others the habit continues unabated when very suggestive reasons for its existence have been revealed ; in yet others there may be a dramatic improvement for no known reason.

Mrs. E. B. a married woman of 29, came to see me with this complaint. It caused her no little embarrassment and had made life a misery for her in the army. She had seen several doctors and had been thoroughly investigated but no cause for the habit had ever been found. Her "nerves" were blamed, but no radical treatment had been attempted.

This patient was one of the most loquacious I had ever come across. No session seemed long enough and in all I saw her eleven times. She was the eldest of a four child family. Her mother died when she was 10, and the family moved to live with her paternal grandmother. Her father was evidently a sadist and she drew graphic pictures of how as a child of 12 she was stripped and thrashed unmercifully with his belt, the punishment ending with her being locked in a dark bedroom to cry her eyes out. She had rather a childish emotional outlook and as she reeled off a succession of these stories I felt they were probably exaggerated. Her next sibling was a sister who had all the looks. Thoughtless relations often pointed this out and told my patient she should have been a boy. She was very surprised when she found an admirer who ultimately married her in spite of her appearance. Here again she was exaggerating. Although no beauty queen she was quite a good looking girl. At the 8th session I managed to guide her back again to discuss her original complaint. She replied that bed wetting was now a thing of the past. She had removed the rubber sheeting from her bed and was confident she was better. I had three more sessions with her but I never discovered the psychopathology of her habit amid the welter of her numerous emotional experiences. Three years have now passed and she has never relapsed.

In the absence of any psychopathology, benzedrine to lower the waking threshold is well worth a trial, and huge doses may be necessary. One child of 12 required 15 mgm of amphetamine before sleep was light enough to be broken by the bladder reflex.

Homosexual Problems

Freud evolved the theory that in infancy a male child is mentally attached to his mother, that is "mother fixated".

By seven years or so the child is veering toward the father and when he is at puberty he should be fixated towards the male and thus homosexual. He looks up to the big boys at school and has ideals in great athletes. It is the age of hero worship. At boarding schools, homosexual practices in the form of mutual masturbation are not uncommon. The fair sex is frowned on, a boy is ashamed to walk with his sister, so great is the taboo on females and all things feminine. At 16 or 17 this phase passes and heterosexual feelings return. The boy begins to take a pride in his appearance. His hair becomes plastered with brilliantine; his tie is put on straight and with care. Female company intrigues and attracts him. All these various phases have divorced him from his mother so that he seeks a mate away from his home. As a child he loved and was protected by his mother; as a man he loves and protects his wife.

The same process happens to girls. At an early age they turn from the mother to the father. A soldier's wife told me how her small girl would talk or play with any man in khaki, but would become quite withdrawn and shy with a strange woman. At puberty girls are homosexual with "crushes" and "grand pashs" and at 17 or so they emerge as mature young women, more mature than men of their own age.

The normal individual passes through all these phases to maturity; but he never completely discards the early bonds of affection. He still retains a trace of mother fixation and the homosexual urge; but these forces should be dominated by the mature heterosexual attitude. Put another way we are all bisexual animals. Most of us have dominant heterosexual feelings; but latently we are also homosexual. A man's love for his wife may, for a time, fill his whole life, but the normal average man enjoys men's company as well. The society of males is different from that of women; and the contrast of company is rather pleasing. Bisexuality is evident in nature. One cow, behaving like a bull, will mount another cow which is in season. This perverted action among cattle is most useful to the farmer, because it shows when his cows are ready for mating.

While most of us are a good mixture of both qualities, there are people who feel no conscious attraction whatever towards the opposite sex and these people are extreme or overt homosexuals. Such people vary in outward appearance. Some are manly figures which one would never suspect of such perversion. Every now and again a famous name in the athletic world becomes prominent in criminal courts when the unfortunate victim of the perversion is found out. Most people express surprise and are deeply shocked to hear that such a manly man should be guilty of such crimes. These unhappy people receive little sympathy for their perversion which is no fault of their own. Other homosexuals have a definite feminine appearance; the typical case overdresses, wears gaudy effeminate clothing, has long hair, is fond of fine silk underclothes, wears rings and a flashy tie pin and so on. He talks and walks in a peculiar way which makes him the butt of the music hall. Any observant man or woman can recognise this type in the extreme case. Among themselves the manly and effeminate type of gross homosexual recognise each other without difficulty. They often form liaisons which are rarely discovered and it is difficult in fact to see that much harm can be done by their activities, illegal though they be. It is serious, however, if the overt homosexual molests and seduces small boys who may thereby be psychologically hurt or even contaminated by the offender. Their crimes then appear to be in line with those of heterosexuals who rape and seduce womenfolk and young girls.

The overt homosexual occurs only rarely compared to the latent types. The latter may be quite unaware of his tendency and the idea of homosexual practices never occurs to him. He will however be lucky if he is not picked out at one time or another by practising homosexuals. This latent group varies widely. It comprises the confirmed bachelor type, the club man, the fellow who runs the scouts and is good with boys, the impotent husband, the habitual drunkard and those with a persecution complex, the paranoid individuals. All bachelors, scoutmasters and drunkards are not necessarily homosexual by any means, but a man's habits and hobbies may suggest such a tendency. This latent homosexuality can produce a surprising range of abnormal behaviour. The absence of normal sexual feelings may be dealt with in two ways. It may be over compensated to produce the Don Juan type who subconsciously fears his own tendencies and tries to convince himself of his manhood by his innumerable conquests. On the other hand, it may be accepted as a virtue, in which case the patient becomes a self righteous prude. One patient, told me how, when he was a young man living in a boarding house, a girl resident had come into his bedroom and made advances to him, and he spoke with obvious pride and pleasure of how he had put her across his knee and spanked her. Later when this patient married, he tried to have his own bedroom, but his wife would not hear of it. He was appalled at the idea of a double bed. He grew accustomed to the idea in time, and in the end he and his wife actually produced a family, in spite of his inhibitions.

The treatment of the overt homosexual is quite beyond the scope of the general practitioner, if indeed anyone can cure such conditions. The complete homosexual never marries, dislikes the intimate company of women and would never of his own free will seek medical or psychiatric advice for his condition. He is quite content with his perverted state. Lesser grades of homosexuality are not always so happy and contented. It is true that many may marry, have children and be good husbands because even the predominantly homosexual is bisexual, but many develop anxiety states or even psychoses as a result of their hidden tendencies and it is then that the problem of homosexuality has a practical issue for the general practitioner. He cannot eradicate homosexual feelings but he can allay anxiety largely by encouraging his patients to let the hetero sexual side of his nature develop. If a man with strong homosexual tendencies is allowed to drift he is likely to remain inverted. If he can be made to realise that he is bisexual and induced to take pains to cultivate the hetero sexual side of his life he is likely to gravitate more towards the norm.

A.T., a man of 24, came to see me in a state of great depression. He felt attracted by men and he was sure he was a sexual pervert, and of course, a social outcast. I found he had been engaged but had broken off his romance because he felt he was not the marrying type. He told me he had enjoyed kissing and caressing his girl and he had actually had intercourse which he had enjoyed. I explained the theory of bisexuality and assured him if he had been a real invert, he would have never reached the stage of getting engaged; he would have avoided female society and he would certainly never have come to me for help. I advised him to seek female society at dances and so on. I assured him that if he sought female company he would encourage the growth of his heterosexual self and perhaps he might find a girl he wanted to marry. I had three sessions with him and when I saw him a year later he told me he had ceased to worry. This man was not of course a true homosexual. He was in an anxiety state because he became conscious of a homosexual tendency which we all of us possess.

A.N. was an army officer of 25. He was sent into our hospital because he had threatened to commit suicide and had been caught playing with a revolver in a suspicious manner.

He was depressed but not markedly so, and gave no history of insomnia. He told me that for two months he had been worried about himself as he thought he had venereal disease. There was in fact no evidence of this. His fear of venereal disease was accounted for by his two experiences. A visit to the medical museum in Cairo had shocked him and filled him with apprehension about the disease and three months prior to my seeing him he had taken a girl out. According to the patient, she had seduced him and he had hated the whole procedure and felt unclean afterwards. He did not like women's company or dancing and he could not think why he should have taken such a risk. Troubles never come singly. Soon after this incident he had trouble with his commanding officer over some trivial routine job. This criticism rankled and he felt resentful, but was powerless to justify himself. The disgrace of "venereal disease" and the rebuke from his commanding officer were too much for him. He admitted he could never stand criticism.

After three sessions of psychotherapy he had lost his fear of venereal disease and I put it to him that his attitude to life was wrong. I suggested frankly that he was immature and had not yet passed the juvenile stage of homosexuality. This was demonstrated by his dislike of women and his repugnance towards the sexual act. I suggested as a counter measure he should seek more female company, and if he took pains to cultivate women friends he would find interest and pleasure in them. It was foolish just to drift, and allow his homosexual nature to dominate the hetero sexual side. I pointed out the latter was there because he would never have been trapped by his seducer if he had not found some attraction. At the end of the interview I asked him if I had offended him by my frank views. "If you had talked like that two weeks ago, I would have thrashed you", he said, "but I think you have only drawn a fair picture of what I am really like." At a later interview he asked me in fun if I could give him any practical hints on how to cultivate the friendship of girls. I felt in spite of his flippancy he was thinking along more healthy lines.

G.L., a man of **27**, was a typical effeminate homosexual. From his flashy gold teeth to his dapper suede shoes he was the caricature of a "cissy". He told me sex had no appeal to him, but life was made a complete misery for him by ridicule and assault. He had been attacked and exposed more times than he could count and in all his jobs, both men and women made fun of him. He was depressed and miserable and wished he was dead. He had refused to go to work, but his family grumbled because he brought in no money. Even his family were against him. He had no friends and no one whom he could trust, a truly paranoid outlook. I held out no hopes for changing him, but felt it might help if he could be placed in a suitable job. I discovered he was an expert at sewing and had made some exquisite embroidery, so rang up the employment exchange where I found the officer in charge most helpful. He interviewed the man and felt as sorry for him as I did. He sent him on a tailoring course at which he is now doing very well. He has the promise of a job in a local firm when he is qualified. The future employer knows the man's difficulties and is prepared to employ him and protect him. Where psychotherapy is impotent to help, sheltered employment may make life useful and tolerable for the complete misfit.

Short Cases

When one has developed confidence in psychotherapy and the psychiatric approach, it is not always necessary to embark on the whole ritual of psychotherapy. From time to time minor cases occur which can be successfully dealt with on the spot. The girl J.B. described in Chapter II is an example. This method is only applicable when the symptoms have only been apparent for a very short time. No long standing case can be dealt with summarily.

M.E. was a girl of seventeen, who complained of sickness and loss of appetite. She had just returned from a seaside holiday and looked a picture of health. I asked her to go upstairs and get ready for an examination, and when she had gone I questioned her mother about her. She was apparently in the midst of packing up to go to college. She had never been away from home; she was the only girl in the family and she had an overprotective mother. I suggested that the queer feeling in her middle was probably due to the apprehension of leaving home. She had simply failed to correlate her feelings with her circumstances. I saw the patient and as I had anticipated I could find no evidence of physical disease under the bronzed skin. I talked about her college and persuaded her to discuss the fears and hopes she had for the future. I told her that leaving home was a wrench, but that she would find her new and emancipated life well worth while. I advised her to write to her mother fully if any problems arose. When I got downstairs the mother said she was sure that I was right. She could remember how bilious M.

had been during her first week at school. The girl has been teaching for a year now and since that interview she has only once reported sick with a septic skin rash. The consultation took half an hour of my time, required no medicine and no further attention.

J.H., a man of 29, came to see me complaining of pain in the lower part of his stomach. I could find no evidence of organic disease but I felt sure he was worried about his appendix.

I told him I could find no evidence of bodily disease, and suggested that worry could easily cause such pains. He assured me he had no worries at all. He had a very capable wife, a nice family and his shop was flourishing. He told me that although he had only been in business for a year, he had made steady progress. There was not much to show in profits because he was ploughing them all back into his business. In five more years he would be well off, he assured me. He talked frankly and eagerly about his ambitions; it was obvious that they were of great importance to him. "What would happen if you had an appendicitis?" I asked him. "That would be a calamity", he exclaimed. He ran a one man business, and if he had to shut up his shop for a month before he was firmly established he would lose a great deal. "Do you still say you have no worries?" I asked. He smiled as he saw my point and he admitted that the fear of developing appendicitis at this crucial period in the build up of his business had worried him a good deal.

I saw him again some weeks later, and he said he was quite better and proceeded to tell me how he had explained to a business friend suffering from indigestion that he was probably worrying too much about his work !

Mrs. A.S., aged 25, was the mother of two small children. She came to see me complaining of a pain in the lower abdomen for which I could find no explanation. The art of psychotherapy is to free the patient from inhibitions and to make her speak her mind. I told her I could find no evidence of serious disease. I then tried to find out what she was afraid of. There was no fear of appendicitis. After a few minutes of conversation, haltingly she told me the real trouble. On the night before her visit to my surgery, for the first time in married life she had had an orgasm. That to her spelt pregnancy and she already had two small children. I explained the wisdom and necessity of contraception to her, and I added I was sure her pain had been caused by the worry she had over pregnancy. A week later she menstruated and she came to tell me the good news. She never had any more vague abdominal pain. This case took in all about half an hour to treat.

The satisfaction such successful short cases give to both the doctor and patient is considerable. It can be compared to the gratification both feel when a foreign body is successfully removed from the eye or behind the finger nail.

REFERENCES

(i) T. A. Ross. The Common Neuroses. 1937.
(ii) **Strän Olsen.** *Lancet,* 1950 (ii) 133.

CHAPTER V

MELANCHOLIA

MELANCHOLIA as its name implies is as old as the history of
medicine. In terms of the Hippocratic humors it was due to
a blackening of the bile. In the middle ages it was a popular
diagnosis, but the absorbing interest of modern internal
medicine in the nineteenth century brought about a partial
eclipse of functional disorders. Depression became a symptom of organic disease and was rarely diagnosed as a separate
entity. Only profound depressions were classified as melancholia. In most mild cases an organic diagnosis was blamed
for the depression. Thus observation of the condition was
largely confined to the precincts of the mental hospitals.
Kraines (i) recently described the situation as follows:—
"Most that is written about this condition is based on the
studies of patients who have become ill enough to be committed to an institution : and there is a dearth of information
about the *vast group** who never enter an institution".

From the surveys given in the first chapter it can be seen
that endogenous depression† or melancholia comes next to the
anxiety states in frequency. No less than 24 per cent of the
psychiatric casualties were due to this condition which
amounts to about 3·0 per cent of all the cases seen in general
practice. It is about as common as joint rheumatism (3·4 per
cent) or all forms of organic heart disease (3·1 per cent). It
is more common than all forms of nervous dyspepsia and the
peptic ulcer syndrome (2·5 per cent). The peptic ulcer syndrome has long been recognised as a major social problem
and vast amounts of time and money have been spent in research on the subject. Endogenous depression is a problem

*Italics ours.

†Synonyms are also primary, or psychotic depression.

of equal importance but it is largely ignored because it is unrecognised. Since the problem is socially so important, and because the condition is so easily misdiagnosed, the subject is discussed in detail in this book.

Symptoms

Endogenous depression is a disease mainly of symptoms, with few reliable physical signs. If one seeks an early diagnosis, or, in mild cases, a diagnosis at all, one must observe the symptoms long before they become the classical triad of difficulty in thinking, depression, and psychomotor retardation.

In all branches of medicine the art lies in early diagnosis. Surgeons tell us that in the early diagnosis of cancer lies the only hope of a cure. Public health authorities encourage us to send our tuberculosis subjects for X-ray and investigation, and no longer expect us to wait for cavity formation before making a diagnosis. If we miss making an early diagnosis in this type of case, we are made painfully aware of our mistakes when the truth becomes apparent. Melancholia, however, is not a killing disease except for the occasional suicide, and the vast majority of cases eventually get better on their own. To wait for the triad of symptoms is like waiting for cavity formation in tuberculosis. If an early diagnosis is to be made, and the patient is to be kept under adequate supervision, the symptoms must be sought in the earliest stages under the following headings :—

    (i) Depression.
    (ii) Suicidal ideas.
    (iii) Changes in the sleep rhythm.
    (iv) Habit changes.
    (v) Pre-delusions : morbid obsessions and phobias.

Depression

Depressed feelings can and do arise in every normal person, in much the same way as healthy people are from time to time afflicted by headaches, indigestion or rheumatic twinges. It is difficult to define a borderline between health and disease. Perhaps it may reasonably be supposed that if a person feels bad enough to come and wait in the doctor's surgery to expound his feelings, he must be considered as ill. His depression has crossed from being an every day ailment compatible with health, and has become a symptom of ill health.

From time to time a typically retarded case may be seen, with obvious difficulty in thinking, and misery written on his face : but far more often the depression has to be sought by observation, listening and a detailed history of the case.

"I'm not really ill, I'm just run down" : "I've just dropped in for a tonic" or "My nerves are all on edge" : these are typical opening remarks which point to depression. Frequently the patient knows he is not physically ill, and blames his nerves. This is just the opposite of an anxiety state, in which the patient usually thinks he is physically ill.

Mrs. F.A., aged 63, came to see me as she felt she wanted a tonic for her nerves. She was upset because her son's wife had left him. This she was sure was the cause of her trouble. Taken at face value this looked like an anxiety state but it was indeed quite a severe grade of depression.

She was slow in her speech and had obvious difficulty in thinking. She was agitated and all the time fiddled and played with her hands, her gloves or her handbag.

With encouragement she talked more, but it was a slow business. She suggested it was her younger unmarried son who worried her most. She feared he would meet the same fate as his elder brother. She distrusted his girl friend though she knew she was wrong and despised herself for it. They were a nice couple really, but she could not help worrying. She would just have to pull herself together, she told me and mumbled on in a slow monotonous voice, with her eyes staring first in one direction then in another, but rarely looking directly at me. She was not given to weeping, but felt like it at times. She had marked insomnia. She denied any wish to be dead—but in such a way that I felt it was not a true answer.

As in venereal disease phobia, undue concern over a trifle may be another typical symptom of depression. One patient came to see me about his cough. He was obviously very concerned about it and indeed appeared to have a troublesome bronchitis. Just before leaving he thrust out his hand, "Look at that", he exclaimed, with a dramatic gesture, and pointed to an insignificant pimple on the dorsum. I mentioned this to my partner after surgery as he had been attending him for some time, and I learned that at his last interview the man had burst into tears. Tearfulness is a common symptom in women and by no means spells severe depression. In women the worse depressions do not cry, they are as it were beyond tears. Crying in a man is more significant and the man who weeps in the surgery is usually depressed to a pathological degree. This unusual show of emotion in a man, coupled with the importance he obviously attached to his trivial pimple and deep concern over his cough, made the diagnosis obvious and the nature of the illness was later confirmed by a psychiatrist.

Another patient insisted that his trouble was entirely due to a quarrel with his foreman. He was obsessed with the idea which he could not get out of his mind and yet he felt physically ill enough to be visiting the doctor. While such an obsession lasts it amounts to an "idée fixe", but it can suddenly change and be forgotten almost overnight or exchanged for a new symptom. This patient appeared one day triumphant; he had discovered what was wrong with himself; he needed new glasses! He had forgotten all about the quarrel.

The depressive is upset by noise. The fond parent is worried and alarmed to find he cannot stand the noise of his children while previously he had revelled in their banter and chatter. The wireless is an almost universal noisemaker and in depression the "wireless test" is usually positive. The woman who used to have the radio blaring all day cannot bear to have it on. The average depressive cannot tolerate the wireless and finds himself switching it off, whereas before he took it as part of the normal background of his home life.

The powers of concentration have gone. Reading is a good measure of this ability. The average case who used to read, cannot finish his books, or forgets what he has read. He can usually read the newspaper. Mrs. F.A. described above could not even read a newspaper.

The ability to enjoy life has gone. Pleasure has lost its sense of satisfaction : beauty has become drab and colourless. A.H. was a keen gardener and grew prize chrysanthemums. Whereas previously he could always spend a happy hour or two in the greenhouse, when depressed he just opened the door looked in and walked out again. Even his most lovely blooms gave him no satisfaction or pleasure. G.I., who was a good type of labourer, was left an unexpected legacy of £4,000. I have never seen a sadder man. He drew no pleasure from his windfall until his depression had cleared. There is a marked falling off of sexual desire. One man told me whereas he had always enjoyed sexual intercourse twice a week, he now rarely had it more than once a month—if that.

Everything is an effort. The housewife has to drive herself to work, and things which she used to take in her stride become major problems of life. Decisions are particularly difficult to make. If a holiday is suggested and a rest from the strain of having to work, there are always a score of excuses. The patient who can barely stand the strain of one situation finds it almost impossible to face another even if it promises relief. Here it is perhaps apt to point out the cruelty of having to add to the difficulties of the patient by suggesting a mental hospital. If to decide on a pleasant change presents difficulties, what concern and alarm must be aroused by such a thoroughly unpleasant decision

In depression time seems to drag. "From tea to bed time seems like two days" one man told me. What an infernal complaint it is ; not only is the suffering extreme, but it is extended by time going so slowly.

Suicidal Ideas

Only the worse cases of depression are frankly suicidal.

Suicidal ideas or the "death wish", as it may be termed, may be classified as follows :—

(a)　No wish to be dead evident.
(b)　No wish to be dead evident ; but the patient is obsessed with the idea that he has a mortal illness.
(c)　The patient is so bad that he wishes he were dead.
(d)　The patient is actually suicidal.

This subject must be approached with tact. One does not want either to upset the patient, or to put ideas into his mind.

If the patient admits depression to me, I ask him if he ever wishes he were dead. Only if he assents do I ask him if suicide has ever crossed his mind. If he admits to this, he usually qualifies his remarks either by saying he is too strong willed to do it, or that his family or his religion give him the strength to resist the urge. A negative reply to the question does not mean there is no suicidal urge. One woman denied any such feelings, but when she had recovered she told me whenever she heard a train coming (a colliery track passed close by her house), she dare not go outside in case she threw herself on the line. Another patient denied suicidal feelings but later admitted he had read a lot about the subject lately and told me a graphic story of how a neighbour "did himself in". When I asked him again about his feelings he admitted he had the urge at times, but cloaked them to save his wife from worrying.

One of my cases having denied ideas of suicide later made an unsuccessful attempt in which she was very cunning.

Mrs. H.A. was a woman of 40. I was urging her to have treatment at a mental hospital, and while waiting for her to make up her mind I gave her amphetamine and barbitone soluble. I was called out urgently one morning as she was in coma. I could rouse her but she was very stuporous. I asked to see her tablets and she still had 5 out of the 7 barbitone tablets. I was puzzled until her husband noticed she had substituted bismuth tablets for the sleeping drugs !*

*Powerful hypnotic tablets should only be prescribed in small numbers, and they should be in the care of relatives who give them to the patient as required.

If the degree of depression is profound it is fairly easy to discuss suicide. The discussion helps the patient as he is relieved to find someone who can share his guilty secret without being shocked. If there is any suspicion of a suicidal urge, the relatives must be informed of this, and once again the subject needs to be tactfully handled. One does not want to panic them, but the need to keep a constant and unobtrusive watch on the patient must be stressed. Actually, if a patient is suicidal, it is surprising how often the relations are aware of it. When the need for watching him is stressed, they reply, "We haven't left him alone for weeks now." Most depressions which are sufficiently profound to have a strong suicidal urge are fairly easy to diagnose, but every so often the diagnosis eludes one. This is especially true if the patient has a clear organic diagnosis which distracts one's attention from the psychological make up.

A patient once called to see me with a septic finger. The condition was aggravated by her wedding ring which had to be removed. She was very silent while this was being performed, and when I asked her if she had ever had it off before she said "No, and I don't like having it off now". I put her remark down to superstition, but 3 weeks later she committed suicide. When I checked up on the case she had made many significant remarks to her friends but no one had noticed she was depressed. I am always on the look out for this condition, but I never spotted or even suspected it in this case.

Insomnia

This is a constant feature of melancholia. The most common form of insomnia is the early waking type, but it is by no means always the case. Typically the melancholic falls off to sleep easily but awakens two or three hours later and sleep has gone for the night. He is restless and depressed and his thoughts consist of morbid ideas which go round and round in his mind. He feels like going to sleep when it is time to get up. Others complain of difficulty in dropping off to sleep ; some sleep fitfully and some are upset by dreams. "I dream of terrible and shameful things", "I never had such dreams in my life", and "I am always dreaming of death and dead people", are examples of how such dreams are described. Sometimes symptoms are blamed for the insomnia. "I could sleep but for my cough", said one patient. Another, who at 53 had a pseudocyesis, could not rest because of "movements".

No matter what the form of insomnia, the patient usually complains of "feeling awful" on waking. The typical mild depressive does not feel bad all the time. He is usually worst in the morning and better by mid-day. By night he may be quite hypomanic. "I can start doing all the work when it's time to go to bed", said one woman. This swing of affect is, of course, typical of this disease. In this illness more than in any other there are good and bad days. The patient will report to the surgery one morning that he has quite recovered, and be in the depths of despair the next. The picture may indeed be a typical manic depressive psychosis in miniature. One man told me with delight how well he felt and how as he had stacked his ton of coal into the shed, he felt strong enough to throw it in in one lump. He found it hard to understand how his moods could alter so quickly.

It must be underlined that insomnia is an essential feature of depression. If the patient says he sleeps well but otherwise seems depressed, it is worth while asking his sleeping partner about his sleeping habits. She may tell a very different story. In a series of 81 cases only one man professed to sleep well, but his wife asserted he was restless at night and was frightening the way he talked in his sleep, although by morning he could remember nothing about it.

Change of Habit

Change of habit in a melancholic may be quite striking. It may be in some general way, such as sociability or in personal hygiene ; or in some special activity. The pianist loses all interest in her piano, the entertainer loses his sense of humour, or the keen amateur gardener lets the weeds grow unheeded. Smoking or alcohol may suddenly be dropped, because they are blamed for the unpleasant symptoms, or drinking may be started in an effort to dispel the unpleasant feelings. One patient of mine went on to delirium tremens as he relied on brandy to get him to sleep, though previously he had always been most abstemious. One old gentleman of 63 had always taken a ritual purge of salts on a Sunday. When depressed he dropped this habit of a life time and when he took it up again, he was on the road to recovery. Psychomotor retardation is usually at the back of habit changes, but the sudden change of habit is often more obvious than the general inhibition.

Phobias, Obsessions, and Delusions

Frank delusions are usually preceded by what may be described as predelusions. These take the form of phobias or obsessions about disease. The patient is convinced he has a cancer, tuberculosis, heart trouble, venereal disease, or that he is going out of his mind. In another form the patient has a kind of dread hanging over him, a feeling that something awful is going to happen, either to himself or to his family. One woman was convinced she was about to have a stroke, and every time she had a queer feeling in her leg she went into a panic. Another woman expressed it by saying, "Every time I hear a car stop, I feel they are bringing my husband back from the mine". Others are fearful for their children and are tense with anxiety until they are safely home from school.

Attacks of panic are not uncommon. The patient is convinced he is about to die. The symptoms must be very distressing and sometimes amount to "angor animi" in which the patient feels dissolution is imminent. These attacks may be accompanied by a rigor. I have seen patients shaking so much that they make the bed rattle and looking like an acute pyogenic blood infection. There is however no temperature and a rapid sedative such as seconal soon relieves the condition. Feelings of unreality are not uncommon, nor is the feeling that the patient is in some way or another unworthy. Their condition is their own fault and a kind of retribution.

Frank delusions are uncommon. In a series of 81 cases collected in general practice I found only 10. These included delusions of poverty and ideas that the patient was wanted by the police ; that the husband did not want his wife any more ; that the patient had committed the unforgivable sin, and so on.

Predelusions are illustrated by the following cases:—

Mrs. E. L., a woman of 46, came to see me with a fissure in ano which had caused her great distress. I gave her a proctocaine injection and when I next saw her she said the pain had gone, but she was still not right. Further probing elucidated severe insomnia, depression with no suicidal ideas and the conviction that she had a rectal growth. There was no evidence of this and I reassured her. I gave her sedatives at night and amphetamine in the mornings but she did not improve. She was still sure she had a cancer. I suggested a second opinion but she refused to take this course. "I am sure you are right now ; but when the feelings come over me I feel certain there *is* something there and I cannot get it out of my mind." The depression cleared in three months and the fear of cancer went with it. When she had recovered she told me she had had severe suicidal feelings but she did not like to admit them at the time.

One of the village fathers, a venerable man of 65, came to ask me for a tonic as he was run down. His symptoms were all very vague and indefinite. Suddenly he said in a low voice, "As a young man I collected venereal disease, 'clap' they called it. This was, of course, before I was married. I have never told a soul that before. I have been wondering lately what my children would say if they knew, or what my friends and their wives would think of me. I know they would have no further dealings with me." I examined him to satisfy him that this was not due to the sins of his youth. His W.R. was negative. I pointed out to him that he had an exceptionally fine family and had done extremely well. This man had started life as a collier and when I saw him he owned a business worth thousands. He remained depressed for about three months and then recovered only to fall victim to a coronary thrombosis. With his physical illness there were no signs of depression.

One man asked me to arrange for him to be castrated and a woman asked to have her womb removed. In the latter case the woman blamed her depressive feelings on her partial prolapse, although she had had her pelvic trouble for years. I dissuaded her from operation and once the depression cleared she lost her pelvic symptoms. Operations never alleviate a depression. Three of my cases who had an operation were all made worse and are now chronic depressives.

G.G. was a woman of 43. I was called in to see her as she was brooding because she was pregnant, her only other child being a girl of 20. She felt she had done wrong to have another baby at her age, and was fearful what people would say, especially her daughter. The daughter knew and said nothing to hurt her mother, but that made no difference to her mother's ideas on the matter. She was agitated and could neither eat nor sleep, and threatened to throw herself downstairs. Her one thought was that she had done wrong to fall pregnant again. Her condition was such that hysterotomy was performed. For a month she was better, but then grew worse than ever. This time she was wrong in that she had done away with her own child. It was an unforgivable sin. After about a year of this state she improved, and I was glad to see the last of her as she would accept no treatment from any specialist or hospital. However in a follow up interview I saw her at her home, and she was as bad as ever in a chronic state of depression.

The other cases who submitted to operation had a hernia and a prolapse and both had been on the waiting list for months. When their admission cards came they were both eager to have the operation and to get better ; but they were worse after the treatment.

All three of these cases were of a poor personality type, so it is unfair to blame operation for the chronicity of their disease, but the point remains that one can expect no amelioration of depression by operation, even if the patient thinks her prolapse or pregnancy is the cause of her symptoms.

Angor animi was shown in the following case:

W.S. was a man of 67. I was called in to see him late one night and I could see from the general consternation that everyone, including the patient, was expecting the worst. He was clasping a hot water bottle to his belly and bidding everyone farewell. I could find no evidence of organic disease. The certainty with which he told me he was finished, his tearfulness and a history of insomnia for 3 months made me diagnose depression. This was in fact the beginning of a chronic depression which 18 months later took him to a mental hospital after he had made a half-hearted attempt to commit suicide in the horse trough. In my experience few patients realise when they are going to die. If they are "sure of it", then it is usually a manifestation of depression.

Presentation of the Disease

The patient may complain of his nerves or difficulty in sleeping, but the presenting symptom is usually quite mundane. In a series of 81 cases the initial complaint was as follows :—

Cough	8	cases.
Feeling run down	7	,,
Depression	6	,,
Headache	5	,,
Vague complaints, indigestion, insomnia .	4	cases for each symptom.
Nervousness, pain in back, tight feelings in chest, belching of wind . . .	3	,, ,,
Vertigo, dysuria, fainting, pregnancy, muscular pains, attempted suicide, strange behaviour, pain in chest, vaginal bleeding	2	,, ,,
Tinnitus, globus hysterious, nettle rash, tremor, rigor, pseudocysesis, bad smell in nose, piles, diarrhœa, collapse, hæmatemesis, fissure in ano . . .	1	,, ,,

If these various headings are consolidated in systems, they would appear as follows :—

Nervous system including psychiatric symptoms . . . 28
Chest and respiratory system 16
Vague complaints 11
Gastrointestinal system 11
Urogenital system 7
Muscular system 5
Skin 1
Ears 1
Collapse 1

    81

Because melancholia not infrequently stimulates organic disease, Kraines (i) coined the phrase "depressive equivalent" to describe it. What appears to be a typical organic lesion, on closer observation turns out to be a true melancholia. A few examples of this form of endogenous depression are as follows:—

Simulating Gastric Carcinoma. T.J., a man aged 52, sent for me one September because he had had a hæmatemesis. I didn't see the blood but he was obviously very ill. He was pale but not exsanguinated and he was very thin. He had a marked anorexia, but no pain whatsoever. I could find no physical signs in his abdomen, but I suspected carcinoma of the stomach as he looked thoroughly cachectic.

As soon as he was fit enough he was sent for an X-ray with negative results.

In November he was a living skeleton. He complained he could not sleep, and felt awful in the mornings. He was morose and could not bring himself to speak to his family. He admitted he was very depressed, and when I asked him if he had wished he was dead he replied, "I have indeed—but I would never have told you had you not asked me". He stated he could still eat nothing before dinner, but felt better by evening. At bed time he felt much better but could not get off to sleep, showing in fact morning depression and evening vigour fairly common in melancholics.

A week later he was very depressed and admitted that but for his family responsibilities he would get out of it. I persuaded him to see a psychiatrist. The latter reported as follows : "This patient has, as you say, a typical involutional depression of something like 12 months' duration. He should have E.C.T. but refuses to go to a mental hospital. His hæmorrhage is indeed difficult to account for, though it did follow vomiting. Did the strain of retching rupture a vessel?"

The patient was very satisfied with this second opinion, although he poured scorn on the idea of a mental hospital, After a year he had recovered sufficiently to go back to work, and he has never missed a day's work since and is better in eating and sleeping.

Simulating Asthma. S.T. was an old man of 84. He sent for me because he was having attacks of nocturnal dyspnœa. I found him setting potatoes in his garden, so he was by no means an invalid. He actually lived alone and cared for himself.

His story was that at 2.0 a.m. he awakened short of breath. He had to get out of bed and open the window and there was no more sleep. I thought he probably had a cardiac asthma, but there was no evidence of either heart or kidney disease. Linctus and cough medicines were ineffective in helping his dyspnœa. He pressed me to let him know the worst, and all his family felt it was the end. The early waking and his deep concern over himself made me suspect depression. I gave him phenobarbitone gr. i each night and once his sleep had returned to normal he improved considerably. Three years have passed since I last saw him professionally, and his progress has been maintained. He walks 3 miles a day and still does for himself in every way.

I have called this case a depression. It was certainly no organic or progressive disease. He had a very fine health record. My view is that this was a very mild depression which fortunately came and went fairly quickly, lasting in all about 2 months. There was no history of asthma, and I never found any evidence of bronchospasm.

Simulating Rectal Growth. B.R. was a man aged 45, who came to see me in February 1947 complaining of diarrhœa. His stools were running from him in the surgery so that I had to send him home, and go there to examine him. There was a history of alternating diarrhœa and constipation with marked loss of weight. Nothing was found on physical examination either P.R. or per abdomen.

He was referred to hospital where investigations were negative, but it was suggested that he should be kept under observation.

A month later when his diarrhœa had ceased he complained of difficulty in falling off to sleep, bad dreams and awakening unrefreshed. He said he felt awful in the mornings and had done so for at least 3 months. Everything was too much trouble, but he denied being depressed. He was irritable at home and his sexual desires had gone.

I referred him to hospital with the suggestion that he was depressed. This view was confirmed by the physician.

By April he was worse, neither eating nor sleeping. In May his wife came to see me. She was very worried about him and was sure he was suicidal. She agreed to his going to a mental hospital, but we could not persuade him to go. Fortunately he began to improve and by July was back at work, having been "on the club" for 5 months. To my follow-up letter he replied he was much better but not completely well. As I have never seen him since November 1947, I take it he has made a fair recovery.

Simulating Intestinal Obstruction. Mrs. H.E. was a woman aged 57, who came to see me in April 1947 complaining of abdominal pain. Physical examination revealed that her abdomen was distended and she presented a picture of subacute obstruction. I sent her to see a surgeon privately and he admitted her to hospital at once and performed a laparotomy—to find no pathology. I saw her again in May when she came out of hospital. All her abdominal symptoms had gone but she complained of insomnia, early waking in character. She was depressed and lacrimose but admitted no death wish. Her memory was bad and she could not stand noise.

She told me she had been very depressed 27 years previously after the death of a child. She had visited the grave thrice daily and once filled a tub in which to drown herself.

A week later she was somewhat better having good days and bad days. She was very worried about her daughter who was separated from her husband. The depression gradually lifted until, when seen in October, she said she would not come again as she was quite well and her recovery appears to have been maintained.

The case is of interest because the depression did not become obvious until after the laparotomy, but it must have given rise to the obstructive signs and symptoms. Autonomic upsets are not infrequent in depressive illness, as shown by sweating, tremors, fainting and even ague.

Simulating Carcinoma of Lung. C.V., a man of 60 who was a chronic bronchitic and always indulged in a few weeks on the club from time to time, came to see me with his old complaint. On this occasion he did not improve and as he had a persistent tachycardia I sent him for X-ray as I suspected the emphysema might be having its effect upon his heart. After the usual delays, a report came back of a suspicious patch at the left apex, probably tubercular. By this time the man was extremely ill, but there was never any physical sign in his chest. He was always thin but he had wasted away. He was profoundly depressed but I felt this was secondary to his general condition. I thought the "patch" might be a primary lung growth, but a second X-ray report ruled that out and suggested the shadow was one of a healed tuberculosis. He was now almost in a coma, and dreadfully ill. There were still no physical signs to account for his condition. His wife then told me this interesting story. Before his present illness he had been very strange. She thought he was getting "the mania".* Normally an indolent man, he was up at 5.0 a.m.

*Relations are often very shrewd in their diagnoses.

working in his garden. He started repairs on his house and set about them with great zeal. He was full of fanciful ideas such as adopting children or taking in boarders. He grew irate when crossed and on one occasion had struck his wife, a thing he had never done before. This clear picture of mania clinched the diagnosis. He was actually almost in a depressive stupor. I sent him off to a mental hospital and a few electro-convulsive treatments soon put him right. He started to eat and sleep soundly and put on weight. The X-ray reports had made me look for an organic diagnosis in what was an obvious severe depression.

This series of case records may well be completed by describing a typical case of mild depression ; the type which tends to be overlooked or misdiagnosed by general practitioners and consultants alike. The patient was well to do, so that I was able to get the diagnosis clinched from every possible angle.

Mrs. B.E. was a woman of 44. In January 1947 her husband sent for me urgently as his wife had fainted. When I got to the house she was lying in a chair, the colour of parchment. I could feel no pulse, but her eyes were rolling round. I gave her coramine and she soon revived, but it was certainly an unpleasant and frightening attack of syncope.

Her husband, who was a man of means, said he had been worried about her for a long time but she would not see a doctor. The next day I called and performed a complete physical examination. I found no abnormality. She told me she had been off colour for some two years and complained of pain in the lower part of her back. When I questioned her more closely she told me she feared she might have a growth in her womb. I had found no pelvic abnormality, but to be quite sure, I sent her to a gynæcologist who gave a negative report.

A careful history of the case showed that apart from 3 or 4 fainting attacks, she had never been ill in her life or had a doctor except when she had had her babies. She was not the neurotic or hypochondriac type. She said she slept well but had horrible dreams of dead people and funerals. She was a very houseproud woman, but found it difficult to keep up her standard. There was no evidence of any death wish.

As time passed her ability to sleep grew worse, and she sufferred from the early waking type of insomnia. Her back pains had gone, and she now complained of indigestion and belched wind. It was now March and her husband was getting tired of her tardy progress. I sent her to a physician who agreed that the case was functional and suggested she should have her teeth out. The physician would not commit himself to a diagnosis of endogenous depression. I therefore sent her in turn to two psychiatrists and they both agreed with my views. One suggested E.C.T. but was not in a position to give the treatment. The other advised observation for a longer period.

The difference of opinion as to treatment was probably due to the fact that psychiatrists rarely see such mild cases. When the patient asked for my views I told her I felt she could safely wait for a month or two and suggested she had her teeth out in the meantime. This was performed in April, by which time she was already on the mend. Slowly her symptoms lifted and by August she said she was back to normal, her depression having lasted some $2\frac{1}{2}$ years.

The fainting attack was incidental to the disease. It may even have been an epileptic attack, but if so it did not improve her depression. Her E.E.G. was in fact negative. She was very mildly depressed and never at any time had a wish to be dead. She felt vaguely unwell, and incapable of doing all she wanted to do. The negative medical history was very important, and the insomnia developing after a period of bad dreams. I had the patient up for psychotherapy, but she had the feel of a depressive, and I thought the only thing to do was to wait. Amphetamine and other euphoriants were without effect, but happily the condition cleared without recourse to more heroic treatment.

Differential Diagnosis

In a profound depression the diagnosis is usually fairly obvious. The patient oozes depression and makes the physician feel sad. In milder cases, as in the anxiety state, the feel of the patient gives a powerful lead as to the diagnosis. The average depressive has to be sought out with care, weighing up shreds of evidence which together clinch the diagnosis. These various pieces of evidence can be summarised under the following headings:—

Do Circumstances Account for the Depression?

The typical endogenous depression, comes as it were, out of the blue. The patient declares, "I have a good husband, a lovely family and a nice home. I have nothing to worry about; why should I be like this?" Not infrequently a reason for depression is thrust at one, but on closer examination it is found to be inadequate. The old man who had the pangs of conscience over venereal disease in his youth was a typical example. Why after 40 years should a man start worrying about such a problem, which had never really caused him anxiety in the interval? Another patient blamed a quarrel with his foreman, but an examination of the evidence showed he was making a mountain out of a molehill.

Does the Patient's Mind Work Logically?

The neurotic mind is essentially logical, but the depressed psychotic mind cannot reason on normal lines. If the presenting symptom is a phobia such as a fear of tuberculosis, the patient cannot be reassured and often suggests the most drastic and unreasonable treatment. Two patients have pleaded to have the offending lung removed. One can usually lessen the tension of an anxiety state quite easily ; but the depressive refuses to be reassured or convinced by argument. He lacks the ability to reason things out, and any attempt to do so does not interest him or actually makes him worse. He is absorbed in his own feelings, unpleasant as they are. He never tires of repeating his symptoms and will repeat the same story over and over again. His mind seems to be working in a groove like a scratched gramophone record. If it moves from one groove it gets into another and the first is apparently forgotten.

What is His Response to the Psychotherapeutic Approach?

The neurotic patient tends to show an active and intellectual interest in his treatment. He comes as it were half way to meet one. The depressive is completely negative towards treatment or even repelled by it. He shows no interest in what the therapist is doing. One must go all the way to meet the depressive. The neurotic is often afraid of mental illness, and happily he can be assured that worry will not cause a mental breakdown. The depressive usually accepts the idea that his trouble is mental, although he stubbornly resists the idea of a mental hospital. In his heart he seems to know there is something wrong in his mind and he bears no resentment. Although he is difficult to arouse, a description of his symptoms seems to give him some flicker of satisfaction. He is often grateful for the diagnosis perhaps because he is glad to find someone who understands him and sympathises with him. He is so often misunderstood.

As a rule an anxiety state feels better after a single interview. He appreciates the rationale of what is going on and is eager to co-operate. The melancholic is much the same when he leaves the surgery as when he entered it. He gets a certain amount of relief from the rapport which should have been established, and that is why he returns. A good rapport is the most important weapon in the treatment of his disease.

Is He Able to Submerge His Worries?

A depression due to anxiety is still capable of being distracted. The reactive depressive laughs heartily at a funny film and can forget his worries in a jolly party. The melancholic cannot be amused. The funny film has no humour for him, and the realisation of this often makes him more depressed. He avoids such distractions and tends to become asocial.

Insomnia

All depressives exhibit some degree of insomnia ; usually of the early waking type.

Suicidal Ideas

The death wish is usually present in some form. Its apparent absence does not altogether preclude the possibility of suicide.

The most common differential diagnosis lies between true melancholia and an anxiety state with depression. Occasionally depression may cover schizophrenia. This type of case is usually severely depressed and needs a psychiatric opinion in any case. His depression is active rather than negative. He is always thrusting his symptoms forward. He will attend the surgery perhaps twice a day and ring up in the interval saying something *must* be done about it. If he carries with him a sense of urgency that is lacking in a true depression, that suggests a schizophrenia with an overlay of depression.

Treatment

The most important factor in the treatment of endogenous depression is to establish a firm rapport. The illness is usually a long one and such rapport may well be the only factor which keeps the patient going when everything else seems hopeless. I like T. A. Ross's comparison of this with the medical attention in typhoid. There was at that time no specific treatment for typhoid, but the physician's role was none the less important and his constant attention gave the sick man confidence and satisfaction. He was like the pilot of a ship, and the patient was the passenger. As long as the sick man could trust and have confidence in the pilot, no storm seemed insuperable.

Fortunately rapport is fairly easy to attain as long as one has a sympathetic ear, patience to hear the same story oft repeated, and confidence in one's diagnosis.

Treatment can be separated into the following headings:—

(a) Psychotherapeutic.
(b) Symptomatic treatment.
(c) Occupational therapy.
(d) Specialist treatment, *i.e.*, E.C.T.
(e) Rehabilitation.

Psychotherapy

The basis of this is reassurance and encouragement. The same ground can be gone over again and again without the patient becoming bored by repetition. He should be assured that his symptoms are due to his illness, and not to any weakness of will or defect in his character. It reassures him to know the illness is a common one, and well understood by the therapist. It is sometimes useful to ask a patient who has recovered to bear one out in one's ideas, and the sick man is often more impressed by the witness of a fellow sufferer, than by anything else. This is especially useful when urging a patient to go into a mental hospital. Those who have been and recovered are very faithful allies, and they can often make the reluctant patient finally decide to take the plunge and have E.C.T.

It is sometimes useful to describe the patient's own feelings to him, by painting the picture of a typical case. The melancholic is helped by realising that here at least is someone who understands ; someone who will listen to him without laughing at his troubles, and without telling him "to pull himself together". He is told instead that he is suffering from one of the most unpleasant types of illness, but things are not so bad as they seem. One of the bright spots in the whole gloomy business is that the clouds do pass. Recovery rates may be slightly exaggerated and the patient told that out of 50 such cases seen in the past year, all but 2 are now better and back at work. He doesn't really believe all this but it does console him to some extent. He must be reassured that in spite of feelings to the contrary, the illness is self-limiting. He can be told his "dash board" instruments are not recording properly, and until accuracy is restored he must depend on those of his doctor and his relations.

No argument will remove a delusion, but there is no need to agree with it. If a woman asserts that her husband doesn't want her any more, she can be assured that it is not true, but it is just the way the illness makes her feel.

Progress is slow and cannot be measured day by day. The

man who complains he is no better should be asked, "Are you the same as you were 6 months ago?" Often he will reply, "I'm better than I was then, thank God".

When improvement does set in one can rejoice with the patient over every good day, but at the same time one has to warn him that he must not be disappointed if he has a few more set backs. It can be explained that when one climbs a mountain and the summit is in view, one often has to descend into a valley before the final climb can be made. Mountain climbing often forms a useful illustration. If the summit seems as far away as ever, when one looks back one can see real progress has been made, as the valley behind looks equally distant.

No effort should be made to probe into the patient's past. If he says he has had venereal disease, he should be told it is a common disease which many better men than he have had. Neither surprise nor shock should be shown at anything he may tell. Try to assure him there is nothing unusual in any symptom. It's just a part of a common and very trying illness.

It is just as important to treat the relations as the patient. They must be told what it is, warned against suicide should such a caution be necessary, and above all warned not to censure the patient. They must avoid telling him it's just a matter of will power, or that his recovery lies in his own hands. They should not agree with his delusions, but they must not ignore them or ridicule them. Indeed, ideally, each spouse should learn to be a therapist to the sick mate.

Symptomatic Treatment

Sleep. Every effort should be made to promote sleep. Phenobarbitone gr.i or gr.ii is rarely adequate. I find barbitone soluble gr.x-gr.viss the best hypnotic. If the effect wears off I switch to the following mixture:

> Potas. bromidi gr.xv
> Chloral hyd. gr.xv
> Tinct opii ♏v

> Syr. tolu q.s.
> Aq chloroformis ad ℥ss.
> Mitte ℥iv.
> Sig. ℥ss o.n.

The small dose of opium does not appear to be habit forming and I don't tell the patient what he is taking. Normal sleep returns in the end, and I know of no case which has become an addict to hypnotics. In any case, epileptics can take phenobarbitone for years without apparent ill effect, so that if a barbiturate had to be taken every night for life, it would do no harm.

Euphoriants. Amphetamine in some form is the best euphoriant I have found up to date. I give 10 mgm in the early morning and a further 10 mgm about 11 a.m. In certain cases this drug is most beneficial, but on the whole its effect is disappointing.

I don't think there is any danger of habit formation except in the aged and then I don't think it matters. Old people often find new vigour in their declining years from a daily dose of the drug. They don't need to have increasing doses and I think the benefit it gives comparable to digitalis in auricular fibrillation.

I feel sure the solution to the problem of this illness will ultimately be a euphoriant which will tide the patient safely over his depression. It will be something as dramatic and efficient as prostigmin in myasthenia. In the meantime we will have to put up with the inadequate treatment which is available, or in severe and prolonged cases, the crude empiric remedy of E.C.T.

Stilbœstrol is most useful in allaying menopausal symptoms, but it in no way eases depressive feelings. In general it may be said that there is no need to withhold any drug which promises to relieve symptoms, merely because the pain is psychogenic. Aspirin compounds may be given to relieve a headache and alkaline powders to allay dyspepsia, and so on.

Occupational Therapy

Some depressives, notably housewives, are able to carry on with their normal duties, at any rate in a modified form. The melancholic is usually better while doing something, as long as the task is not too arduous, and the patient does not expect too much of himself. A proportion of male patients are able to carry on with work away from their homes, but most have to be put off work. As always one must try to steer the hard middle course between the extremes of attempting too much thereby increasing exhaustion, and doing too little thereby giving the patient time in which to brood. The man off work should be encouraged to do things with his hands and to be sociable with his friends. The purpose of occupational therapy is twofold. It helps to while away the time until the depression is relieved, and it induces a sense of achievement. The depressive always feels so useless; he feels encouraged to find he can do even small jobs.

Electroconvulsive Therapy

This form of treatment is beyond the scope of the general practitioner. It is however the treatment of choice in endogenous depression, as it cuts short the illness by months. Sargant and Slater (ii) suggest it is most dramatic in involutional melancholia where 70–90 per cent recovery can be expected. Tod and Daly (iii) make the figure 46 per cent when it covers all forms of depression. Sands and Sargant (iv) maintain it should be used in depressions of later life, but their oldest case was only 65.

So far as I know this treatment has been largely applied to melancholics who have been bad enough to go to a mental hospital, but it has not been applied to many of the mild cases such as I have described.

I am not in a position to discuss the merits or demerits of the treatment. There are still those who decry it, but psychiatrists as a whole have accepted it as the best form of treatment available for depressives today. Mallinson (v) summed up the matter as follows:—"At the present time it can be said that very few psychiatrists who were called upon to treat mental patients before the introduction of convulsive treatment, and who have now had any experience of E.C.T., would consent to work in a clinic where it was not available".

The domiciliary treatment of endogenous depression is inadequate in three-eighths of the cases. There is usually considerable difficulty in persuading mild cases to go to a mental hospital for treatment. Few melancholics resent the diagnosis of mental illness but most strongly object to the idea of a mental hospital; and so do their relations. The responsibility of caring for such cases without specialist help casts an unfair burden on the general practitioner.

It is not the task of the general practitioner to give E.C.T. but he has to decide which cases should be referred to a psychiatrist. With the severe cases it is obvious, but with the milder ones the decision is more difficult and no one as yet knows the answer. The psychiatrists rarely see early mild cases and the general practitioners are often reluctant to refer such cases even if diagnosed to a mental hospital for treatment, especially as most cases recover on their own in time. I allow my mild cases three months and if there is no evidence of real improvement I pass them on to a psychiatrist. It is not advisable to leave even mild cases indefinitely, as after a year or two they tend to become permanent hypochondriacs, and E.C.T. then has little or no effect.

H.V., aged 49, came to see me with a mild depression which I thought was endogenous in type. As it did not clear I sent him as a voluntary patient to a mental hospital. He was kept under observation and it was decided that his depression was secondary to a peptic ulcer which had troubled him. After three weeks he came home somewhat improved but he soon relapsed. He was very graphic in describing his feelings. At a variety show he could not laugh or see the humour in the jokes which appealed to everyone. He always backed a horse at the weekend, and while he still put his shilling on, he couldn't even be bothered to look at the evening paper when it came. He refused to return to the mental hospital, but when out patient E.C.T. started at the local general hospital he went there for treatment. The psychiatrist now agreed that the depression was endogenous and E.C.T. was given. He had been depressed for some eighteen months by this time, and the result was not very satisfactory. He is still off work and reluctant to start, and before his illness he had a good work record. No accurate assessment can be made on a case like this, but in my opinion if the depressive does not show clear signs of improvement at the end of three months, something more drastic than domiciliary treatment is needed. No promise of out patient treatment should be made, because some cases, even if mild, do better in hospital and they may refuse admission if out patient treatment has been advocated. The best prognosis occurs in patients with a good personality and a good work record. The patient who is always in the doctor's surgery with vague complaints, and frequently on the club, is a poor subject for out patient E.C.T. Hospital discipline combined with E.C.T. offers the best hope of recovery.

Rehabilitation

It is only in recent years that rehabilitation centres have become available. They are an ideal stepping stone to complete recovery for the patient who is left with a feeling of inadequacy and a fear of starting back on his old job. Two brothers, who both had E.C.T. for their melancholia, were left feeling unable to take the plunge back to their old occupations. They were sent for three months to the local rehabilitation centre, and since their discharge they have both been back at work and have ceased to visit me at the surgery. One was off work two years and the other fifteen months. Rehabilitation also works by being a weapon of coercion. F.H. was a man of 45. He had the physique and the mental capacity of a gorilla. He was illiterate and a true moron. After a head injury he became the complete depressed hypochondriac and I never thought he would work again. The labour authorities suggested rehabilitation and as I felt sure he would only waste valuable accommodation at the centre I was reluctant to send him. However, he went, improved up to a point, and returned to light work. He was ill more than at work, and in the end I suggested another course of rehabilitation. This he did not want to undertake. When I gave him a choice of rehabilitation or work, he chose the latter, and so in his case rehabilitation has indirectly served a very useful purpose.

Discussion

Early in this chapter the incidence of melancholia was compared with that of organic diseases. In my experience it is as common as the rheumatic conditions or organic heart disease, and amounts over a period of three years to about 3·3 per cent of all cases seen. This is only part of the story. A follow up of 81 cases showed that the duration of the illness amounted, in those who recovered, to an average of 10 months. In the working man this implied 4 months of complete incapacity for work and six months substandard work. Many cases do not recover but drift into a chronic state of depressive hypochondriasis. Twenty such cases were collected, and they are indeed a problem. Socially they are a complete loss and draw their sick pay month after month until it becomes the old age pension. From the family point of view they are a great burden bringing an atmosphere of gloom and depression into the whole household. Medically they waste more of the doctors' time than most people. They are always with us. They bring with them to the surgery an aura of misery, and there is nothing one can do to help. They can live for years full of symptoms for which there is no apparent cause and no known cure. One patient has seen the doctor at least every fortnight for the last 30 years and what an unsatisfactory consultation it is. Chronic depression was the end result of 12 per cent of all the melancholias seen in general practice. It is a grim fate.

We in general practice may make some rough estimate of the numerical incidence of the disease, but we cannot offer a remedy. It is a serious problem which must be studied by specialist and general practitioner together. In one way the severe depressive is fortunate. His condition is obvious, and if severe enough he is forced to take sanctuary in a mental hospital where adequate treatment is given to him. The mild depression frequently passes unrecognised and even if it is spotted, E.C.T. seems a severe remedy for a mild case. Treatment is put off and evaded by both doctor and patient for as long as possible. Sometimes the delay is too long, and E.C.T. in the end is useless. Depression like schizophrenia needs adequate supervision and treatment in the early stages. If it is slow and insidious in onset, it may pass into the permanent and chronic state before anyone has realised the true nature of the disease. Such a fate rarely overtakes the acute or profound depression which forces one to take heroic action.

In the treatment of anxiety states, the general practitioner can do most of the work himself. With melancholia he must have access to a psychiatrist for a large proportion of cases. In this sphere of medicine there is a great need for close co-operation between the general practitioner and the consultant.

REFERENCES

(i) KRAINES, S. H. The Therapy of Neuroses and Psychoses. 1943.
(ii) SARGANT, W., and SLATER, E. Physical Methods of Treatment in Psychiatry. 1944.
(iii) TOD, H., and DALY, B. G. *Edin. M.J.*, 50, 641.
(iv) SANDS, D. E., and SARGANT, W. *B.M.J.*, 1942, I, 520.
(v) MALLINSON, W. P. *B.M.J.*, 1948, II, 641.

CHAPTER VI

NEUROTIC AND PSYCHOTIC GRAFTS

It is perhaps an adage that there is no such thing as a pure functional ailment, or a pure organic disease. The psyche affects the soma and vice versa. On the other hand from a practical point of view one can divide cases into those which are organic, psychiatric and those which are a mixture of both. This last group include the vast realm of psychosomatic disorders which consist of such conditions as the peptic ulcer syndrome, asthma, rheumatic diseases, thyrotoxicosis, dysmenorrhœa and many problems in gynæcology. While most doctors will agree that there is an important psychological element in these diseases, the problem is most complex, and the treatment of them by psychological approach is usually beyond the scope of the general practitioner. The psychopathology is too deeply hidden in the subconscious to be affected by superficial therapy, and the time factor precludes the lengthy treatment which would be necessary.

The neurotic or psychotic is not immune from a physical illness, and conversely a patient suffering from a frank organic disease may develop some psychiatric illness. It is this small group, a true mixture of functional and organic, which it is intended to discuss in this chapter.

When a neurotic develops a serious organic illness, the neurosis often fades away like summer mists before the sun.

V.S., a man of 26, was very worried about his attitude to sex. He was a Don Juan and had more conquests than he could count. While he could not abstain from sexual athletics, his experiences always left him with depressing feelings of guilt. He was obsessed with the idea that he was sexually abnormal and kept brooding over his fears. A case of this type was referred to in Chapter IV. He was a latent homosexual with a masculine protest. Homosexuals were always picking him out and making advances which repulsed him. In order to prove to himself that he really was a man, he became a "lady killer" and to a certain extent his conquests gave him reassurance. This is not the type of case one would try to treat in general practice. Soon after I had started explorative psychotherapy he developed a virus pneumonia. He became very ill, but in spite of his physical complaint he was delighted with himself. He told me with confidence that he had never felt better, and that all his sexual worries had left him. Unfortunately such relief is usually only temporary, and the neurosis returns as soon as the physical disease clears.

Mrs. G.A., aged 49, was suffering from an apparent endogenous depression. She was miserable and wept a good deal. She wished she was dead and out of the way. She could not sleep at nights, and she was deluded in that she felt she was far gone in pregnancy although there was no evidence to that effect.

I was called out to see her early one morning. She was blue and dyspnœic, with a copious frothy sputum and a severe pain in the chest. I diagnosed a coronary artery thrombosis and treated her with morphia. She was extremely ill, but no longer felt depressed. She felt better once the chest pain had gone than she had felt for months and wondered why she had thought she was pregnant. However, as soon as she was allowed to get up and do odd jobs about the house, she became depressed again, but this time the depression cleared after a few weeks of convalescence.

These are extreme cases, but there must be parallels in the experience of all established practitioners. The old chronic neurotic who is a real burden to attend breaks her leg and at once the visits become quite a pleasure. The patient is cheerful and uncomplaining until she is better physically, when alas, all her hypochondriacal symptoms return.

An explanation for this is very simple if the fact of a purpose in the neurosis is borne in mind. If that purpose is one of attracting sympathy and attention, physical illness does this more effectively and the neurosis becomes redundant. In the same way the neurosis may be an expression of the patient's inability to cope with his environment, and if physical disaster drives him to bed, he is for the time being relieved of this struggle and so the neurosis disappears. Davies and Wilson (i) describe this graphically in respect of hæmatemesis, when often the patient previously worried and harassed declares that he feels better after the calamity. "Wounded in the battle of life, there is an armistice, and with it there is the possibility of a new orientation. The cares and worries of yesterday now seem relatively unimportant." This euphoria comes when an honourable wound has been sustained, one which is obvious to all and which the patient feels he can bear with dignity and courage, attributes which he feels himself were sadly lacking in his normal struggle with environment. The same phenomenon was noticed in the first world war, when it was observed that men with simple "blighty wounds" never developed shell shock. The wound was honourable and even more certain of effecting escape from an intolerable environment than a neurosis.

Physical illness besides rescuing a patient from insoluble problems offers him in return the security of a bed and all the benefits of regression to infantile dependence on others ; a positive force of attraction to the neurotic and especially the immature types which are basically hysterical.*

There is no denying that most of us do enjoy for a time the situation in which we are no longer responsible for the smallest item in our environment. We can relax as dependent children in the care of good parents, and the immature type who is constantly refusing the responsibilities of adult life naturally finds intense satisfaction in returning to the state of infantile dependence. While "his nerves were bad", people were always getting at him, telling him to pull himself together. His complaints never gave complete satisfaction because in one way or another people were always questioning their validity. But once a frank organic disease has descended on him

*Casson ably describes this process of regression. Lancet, 1949, ii, 681.

he is like a man who has recovered his lost passport which gives him the right to live for a while in the land of his heart's desire. This process of regression explains why most people prefer a male doctor who is a good father substitute; while most of us shrink from the idea of a male nurse. A mother substitute for the nursing side of illness has a far greater appeal.

Whatever the mechanism, physical disease imposed on a neurosis often relieves the neurotic symptoms, at least temporarily ; and for the time being the doctor is relieved of having to deal with a double pathology. If however a patient with a physical complaint develops a neurosis, the picture is very different. The neurotic or psychotic graft has indeed a very adverse effect upon the patient's progress. If a complete and normal recovery is to be accomplished, both mind and body must have their full share of attention.

My notice was first drawn to this in a youth of 20 who had a severe cystitis which failed to respond to the usual remedies. The patient was always miserable and in tears and appeared to have a very low pain threshold. I saw him alone and discussed things with him. He admitted a sexual indiscretion and feared his troubles were a just retribution for his sins. He hated his relations to visit him, especially his sisters, as he felt polluted and unclean. A simple explanation of the true pathology, and a reassurance that his troubles was neither venereal disease nor divine retribution went far to relieve his anxiety and physical improvement set in.

Mrs. C.F., a woman of 35 with 3 children, was somewhat similar. She had a pyelitis which readily responded to treatment, and even when the urine was clear and her temperature normal, she looked ill and complained of extreme lethargy and inability to do her work. One day I spent half an hour with her exploring the background of the case. I discovered her mother and sister had died of pulmonary tuberculosis and her brother had died of renal tuberculosis. She admitted she had always dreaded kidney disease, in case she was like her brother. I was able to reassure her on that point and she soon returned to normal.

In both these cases a neurotic graft in the form of an anxiety state was present and sufficiently strong to hold up physical recovery when the physical basis of the illness had been removed. Such neurotic grafts being usually of recent development are fairly easy to remove and the small amount of time necessary for their treatment is quickly retrieved by the early termination of routine visits.

In other cases the neurotic graft may aggravate symptoms which have a physical basis which in itself cannot be relieved. The neurotic and physical symptoms together may produce a marked degree of invalidism, but once the neurotic side of the illness is treated a great improvement in condition is achieved.

Mrs. G.F., aged 45, came to see me complaining of shortness of breath and insomnia. She could not walk more than 200 yards along the level without stopping. At the outset I suspected an effort syndrome, but on physical examination I found that exercise produced a rapid auricular fibrillation and obvious embarrassment. There was no evidence of cardiac failure. I told her that there was some trouble with her heart but I did not think it was serious, and there was no evidence that her heart would let her down. I told her that if she tried to climb mountains or swim the channel she would soon be in trouble. At the same time I told her it would be equally foolish to "wrap herself up in cotton wool". An invalid life would be boring and was quite unnecessary. She was told to steer a middle course and do what she liked as long as it implied no excessive exertion. She came to see me two weeks later and told me she was much better. She could sleep well and could walk a level mile with comfort. In this case there was an overlay of anxiety which I was able to remove and so increase her general efficiency. I saw her two years later suffering from uterine fibroids which have recently been removed, but she has had no further cardiac symptoms.

Such a case underlines the importance of telling the patient the truth in words she can understand. In this case the patient's fears were actually confirmed, but by putting her complaint into its proper perspective, it was possible to remove the associated anxiety.

The following case of neurotic graft also demonstrates the principle that the mind as well as the body sometimes needs attention.

Mrs. S.G., a woman of 36, came to see me with a lump in her neck. I knew she was an anxiety prone individual. The mass looked like a simple septic gland following tonsillitis, but instead of responding to treatment it became larger. A second opinion was suggested and she became panic stricken. She was sure the lump was some deadly disease, and she dreaded seeing a surgeon. She was quite sure she could never stand an operation. She was persuaded to see a consultant and he skilfully coaxed her into hospital where the gland was removed. It was tubercular. When she came home she was still in a great state of agitation and far from well. She was horrified when I told her the diagnosis and begged me not to say any more. However I insisted on explaining the difference between glandular and pulmonary tuberculosis. I persuaded her to come and see me for regular sessions. She had been neurotic long before the gland trouble. She was afraid to be on her own and had a great fear of death. If any relation or neighbour died she was filled with worry and anxiety and was sure she would soon die too. Her mind was full of morbid ideas as to what her husband and children would do without her.

She was the elder of two girls. When her sister arrived she was only two and her maternal grandparents adopted her. She was strictly brought up but had more and better toys than her sister. She was fond of her mother but feared her father. As he drank and smoked, her puritanical grandparents painted him as the epitome of evil, a quite libellous description of him. He was in fact a very ordinary but decent type of working class man. If the patient misbehaved she was threatened by such sayings as "Satan will get you" or "I will send you back to your father" and both became synonymous. She never got on well with her sister, who not only possessed the parents, but who also had more liberty than my patient. This jealousy and hatred was brought out in later years by an unfortunate accident. The patient was then a married woman and well on in pregnancy. Her sister entered the house quietly and gave my patient a fearful fright. She came in to labour the next day but the child was stillborn. She swore she never felt movements after that fright and she blamed her sister for killing her child. "I can never forgive her for that", was her attitude, although obviously the sister had not intended to frighten her. This hatred of the sister was also underlined by dreams in which the rival died.

Fear of dying was linked up with her insecure childhood, and a very real fear of the Devil himself. At the tenth session she revealed an important clue which she had unconsciously repressed ; a clue I should have known about at the start. There was apparently a third sister 4 years younger than my patient who died of a fulminating meningitis at 11 years of age. As one would expect, this child had all the love and affection which she denied her rival sister, and her sudden death was a serious blow to her. However, most of her feelings of sorrow and bereavement were too painful and thus repressed. While she could remember lurid details of her grandmother's death and other family upsets, her conscious knowledge of this great loss was very vague. When I expressed surprise at this omission she said she could not think why she never told me. This incident offered a possible explanation for her fear of death, especially sudden death.

During psychotherapy she expressed a good deal of hatred against her grandparents who had misled her, and her mother who had forsaken her. She spoke lovingly of her father who was in reality kindness itself to her. Discussion about the importance of digging up the past ; of facing one's fears openly and so on, have greatly relieved her anxiety. She is still under treatment but her husband tells me she is much easier to live with and she has lost all her fear of her neck operation and its implications.

In no branch of medicine is a proper psychiatric sense more useful than in gynæcology. Snaith and Ridley (ii) underlined this need in their admirable article on gynæcological psychiatry. The writers pointed out that many pelvic conditions such as dysmenorrhœa, sterility, abortion, dyspareunia and even prolapse have psychological causes in whole or in part. They stressed the importance of assessing both aspects of any such condition, and the need for co-operation between the psychiatrist and the surgeon. Compromise, they suggested was often necessary. "The psychiatrist must always have the courage to give up, at the right moment, his hopes of healing the patient psychically whenever a gynæcologist can eliminate an important defect more quickly ; and the gynæcologist must be prepared to withhold his knife and even his hormones when the psychiatrist suggests that their use may have bad psychological results. He must be prepared to operate on some occasions, even in the absence of demonstrable organic diseases, if his colleague can be reasonably sure that only the removal of the uterus or repair of the pelvic floor will finally reassure the patient and abolish her anxiety state."

It was pointed out in a previous chapter that operation was a bad risk in endogenous depression. This is not so in anxiety states, but the patient does need combined therapy.

Mrs. G.A. was a woman of 38. The list of her symptoms was extensive. She had never been well since she was 17. The outlook for psychotherapy seemed bleak. Her main complaints were a fear of going out alone and dysmenorrhœa, but she also had aches and pains in every part of her body. Menstruation had become painful round about 17, but for the last two years it had grown progressively worse and harder to bear. Her case history showed that at 18 she had lost her mother from pulmonary tuberculosis and, as the eldest of seven siblings, she ran the house for her father. The whole experience precipitated her neurosis. She had nursed her mother during her illness and lost her and as she had a strong bias to her mother, her sense of loss was considerable. She developed an intense fear of tuberculosis and at 18 she was overwhelmed by family responsibilities. At 23 she married and left home. Like many young women who have had to cater for younger siblings, she wanted no family of her own. It was only of recent years she had begun to think in terms of a family; but she felt she was too ill to have one. As I came to know her better she laid more and more stress on her dysmenorrhœa. She said the pains were so fearful she would rather die than face another period. I sent her to a gynæcologist who suggested she might have an endometriosis and that she should be investigated. Preliminary investigations were negative but as pethidine in large doses was the only drug which gave relief, she had a hysterectomy. The uterus was normal. After operation she felt weak and was still fearful of going out alone. She was persuaded to go out for walks, at first with her husband and then on her own. A holiday was suggested and after a fortnight at the sea she felt much better. She was persuaded to try her work again. I last saw her two years ago, when she told me she did not know it was possible to feel so well.

It might be argued that all she needed was a hysterectomy and that the surgeon's knife had cured her. However he had removed an apparently normal organ and the generalised anxiety, with fear of being alone, long predated the severe dysmenorrhœa. She had never really resigned herself to her mother's death, hence her fear of being alone. On marrying she was glad to be rid of overwhelming family responsibilities, and was determined to have no children of her own. Of later years roughly co-incident with the severe dysmenorrhœa, she felt she had missed something by having no family. She wanted an infant but dare not have one, as she was too ill. Her mind was in a state of conflict, and anxiety was concentrated on her pelvic organs. Discussion of her past, her sense of loss, her fear of tuberculosis, and the difficult times she had coping with her siblings, relieved her anxiety but not the dysmenorrhœa. Only the surgeon's knife could do that. The convalescence heralded a temporary return of her anxiety but this was dispelled by further encouragement and psychotherapy. The end result was most satisfactory. Perhaps I am biassed in feeling that psychotherapy played a part in this recovery, but the gynæcologist who directed the surgical side was in full accord with my views.

Psychotic Grafts

Psychotic grafts are quite as common as their neurotic counterparts and they are much more trying to handle. The most frequent trouble of this nature is depression. It is common after such infections as influenza and sinusitis. The patient is miserable and depressed even to the point of suicide. Psychotherapy is quite ineffective and the only course to take is one of observation and reassurance as with endogenous depression.

E.D. was an old lady of 84 of exceptional personality and ability. She lived alone and did all her own housework. In August 1947 I was called out to see her in the night as she had an attack of renal colic. I gave her morphia and the next day she was much better. I noticed she had auricular fibrillation and a fast pulse, so I kept her in bed. She developed œdema and became seriously ill. Her son took her to his own home and there she became very depressed. She did not weep, but she felt she was finished, and she actually asked me to put her away. She could neither eat nor sleep and it was difficult to control her œdema. She had Vitamin B complex as well as her digitalis but her heart condition was a great source of worry to me. Slowly she improved but she remained profoundly depressed. In ordinary times she knitted, did the *Telegraph* crossword puzzle every day and enjoyed jig-saw puzzles, but she could settle to none of these things. She even lost interest in her own home, and she had always been of a very independent nature. Just after Christmas she was persuaded to go away to her other son for six weeks. She hated every minute of the change and must have been a very difficult guest. The doctor who looked after her wrote and told me that while her fibrillation was under control, she was very much a "cracked pot". However she came home in

February and I could see a big improvement. She had started knitting and listening to the wireless. By Easter she was well enough to go home and take up her life again, including her crossword puzzles. From that time until her death from a stroke two years later I had no occasion to visit her except socially. The case itself was very encouraging. No matter how bad the prognosis appears to be in these depressed cases, until the patient actually dies, there is always a hope of recovery. Personality is a great ally in the struggle, and this old lady was of the best material.

Chronic illness is frequently accompanied by periodic depressions. While the melancholia may in fact be due to the monotony and restrictions of invalidism, the attack has the character of a true endogenous depression.

In my opinion few chronic sick are more cheerful in adversity than the victims of chronic rheumatism.

T.W. was a young man of 27 who had been confined to his bed for seven years with a poker back and ankylosing arthritis of both hips. He was usually cheerful and contented in spite of his crippling and sometimes painful complaint. He seemed to have accepted the bad prognosis and adjusted himself to the limited little world in which he was compelled to live. He revelled in the praise he got from his family and friends for his uncomplaining attitude. His bedside became a social centre. But periodically a cloud descended and the patient lost his tranquil frame of mind. He grew restless and demanded further investigation of his condition or a new treatment. He became complaining, morose, and difficult to live with. He felt his life in his deplorable state was not worth living, and suicidal ideas were not far away. He was broody and had difficulty in sleeping. He refused to eat, was depressed and at times lacrimose. He was full of symptoms and each new pain had an ominous significance. His whole attitude to his suffering became illogical and quite the reverse of his usual fortitude.

I only saw this man in one of his attacks but my partner, who has been looking after him ever since his illness began, says he has had three or four similar attacks. They usually last for about a month, and then the cloud lifts and he becomes his old self again, seemingly adjusted to his physical limitations.

G.M. was a man of 64 with a very severe chronic bronchitis and marked emphysema. Only on his best days could he walk very slowly along the village street. Most of his life was spent in his chair in the kitchen. He was a man of character. Starting life as a collier, he had continued at that work until his chest had stopped him five years previously. But besides his mining he had saved money and bought property. He was a fine gardener and owned a sizeable poultry farm. He was always an interesting man to visit, although he was so short of breath that even speech was difficult at times. He was philosophical about his illness, and usually said little about it. He preferred to talk about gardening or hens.

When I called to see him in March 1946 he had left his place in the kitchen and was sitting in a chair in his downstairs bedroom. He looked thoroughly miserable and depressed. He felt his end had come, and although he had no idea of suicide, he wished he could die. Life was a burden to him and he could see no future. His sleep was bad as he was given to early waking. He made a good response to luminal and benzedrine and in about 3 weeks the cloud had passed. He came back to the kitchen and was his old cheerful self until he died in an emphysematous crisis some 8 months later.

When he was feeling well, he told me that for some years he had always got depressed in the spring.

The domiciliary treatment of depression has already been dealt with. These unhappy people need encouragement. So often they think they are alone in their world of misery, it helps them if one can say one has had similar cases before which have recovered. Nevertheless it must be admitted that a depressive graft in an elderly patient is a serious symptom. Loss of appetite readily lends to a lowering of the general condition and a terminal broncho pneumonia often carries the patient away.

In general practice more than in any other branch of medicine, one has the opportunity to view the patient as a whole. Knowing his patients as individuals the general practitioner is especially well equipped to notice any change in the patient's bearing or state of mind. The recognition and, if possible, the treatment of graft accelerates the patient's recovery and will save the practitioner considerable anxiety during the course of treatment, if he realises he is up against a double pathology. The ancient physician of India, Susruta, epitomised the situation in his aphorism: "He that knoweth but one branch of his art, is like a bird with one wing".

REFERENCES

(i) D. T. DAVIES and A. T. M. WILSON. *Lancet*, 1939, II, 723.
(ii) L. SNAITH and B. RIDLEY. *B.M.J.*, 1948, II, 418.

CHAPTER VII

NEUROSES IN CHILDHOOD

THE commonest causes of anxiety among adults were found
to be frustration and insecurity. These forces are often
evident in the environment of a child. The infant's field of
controlled activity is so much larger than that of the adult,
it is at times almost all inclusive, and there is ample room for
frustration. The child is also so dependent on his parents,
and adults in general, so fragile are his growing roots in
society, that a sense of insecurity can readily be produced.

The picture of a childhood neurosis differs somewhat from
the adult prototype. Somatic dysfunction is most common
among adults, but in children it is rare and it is expressed
somewhat differently. Most children pretend to be ill at one
time or another. If one member of the family gets special
attention because of a sore throat or a bad ear, there is a
tendency for the other to try it on. This is, of course, childish
imitation and not a neurosis. On the other hand if the parents
are neurotic and openly pay too much attention to their
subjective feelings, the child does likewise and is on the way
to becoming an introspective neurotic. Symptoms such as
headache, dyspepsia or vomiting can occur in childhood
anxiety, but the manifestations are usually motor rather than
visceral such as tics, mannerisms, or stammering. Anxiety
with depression is comparatively rare, but fears of the dark,
of being alone, of fire and so on are common. These, of course,
compare with adult phobias. In addition, children express
anxiety by a display of aggression or destructiveness which
would be a serious symptom in an adult. The normal grown-
up has learned to control aggression because there are social
limits to its expression. The child has not learned about these
limits nor the power of control. The emotions of a child are
volatile and easily change. In an adult they move much more

slowly and care is taken not to give obvious expression to such changes. When a parent has done something to please a child, the latter will say "I love you, and when I grow up I will marry you". When bed is suggested a moment later, there is a scene and the child exclaims with feeling, "If you put me to bed now, I will never speak to you again ever". Adults rarely come to the surgery because they are troubled with bad dreams, but nightmares in childhood is often the presenting symptom for which the child is brought to the doctor.

It may seem inappropriate to bring a small child to the doctor because he bites his nails, is given to crying or he is afraid of the dark, or because he has tipped the baby out of the pram. Some of us feel baffled and irritated by such problems, and we feel that these habits or actions are within the parents' own province to cure by persuasion or if necessary by force. Nightmares may be explained away by a heavy evening meal but all too often for our peace of mind we detect a note of sincerity in the mother's declaration that nothing unusual was eaten for supper before such attacks. There is in fact very little we as general practitioners can do for these behaviour problems, unless we accept the thesis that they are an expression of anxiety in a child, and the rational treatment is to get down to tracing the origin of the anxiety in each particular case.

Play therapy and a direct approach to the child's problem through contact with the child himself is not possible in general practice. The parents have more time to observe the child and they must be taught enough psychology to find out the cause of the trouble and to lessen the tension. In other words as far as general practice is concerned, the parents, the doctor, and sometimes the teacher, all work together to discover the problem in the child's mind. Once this is discovered attempts must be made to remove it or explain it. In childhood neurosis, circumstances are made to fit the child, rather more often than an attempt made to change the child's attitude.

The mother who is intelligent enough to bring her child for an opinion, readily accepts the idea that the child is nervous, if she has not already come to that conclusion on her own. It is then explained that nerves are due to worry and anxiety and that the child is unable or unwilling to disclose his problem. Such direct questions as "Why are you crying?" or "What frightens you in the dark?" will meet with no useful explanation. The real problem must be sought by a careful observation of the child's behaviour as a whole. I find the following basic ideas of a child psychology interest the parents, give them some ideas as to possible problems and encourage them in their search for the basic cause.

The Mind of a Child

Children live in a world of make-believe. They believe implicitly in certain ideas which are entirely mythical, but these "infantile delusions" serve the useful and essential function of forming a scaffolding which permits proper growth towards maturity. This scaffolding is temporary only and must in its proper time be removed. If it is removed too soon or left too long, the individual suffers in consequence.

The first delusion of infancy is the idea of "all importance". To the small child, he himself forms the centre of the universe, and everything revolves round him. The idea is not altogether a delusion, as a baby is, in a sense, the ruler of the household. The first born child has two parents who are his servants. He realises he is the object of great love and devotion. The sense of personal importance is often portrayed in the child's speech. If he hears his parents discussing the illness of a friend, he remarks "He must have caught *my* cold", because it seems to him that everything happening in the outside world must be related to him. This age of omnipotence is normally ended by the advent of a new baby, or in the case of an only child, by going to school and becoming "a new boy", a very inferior creature among a crowd of potential equals. Both experiences can be very distressing to the child. Most parents prepare the child for the advent of a new brother or sister, but it is very difficult to enter into the child's mind, and the picture an adult passes on to the child is often incomplete and misleading. One small girl was very angry and disgusted with the new baby because he could not play with her, when she had been promised a "little playmate". Moreover she could not, of course, be satisfied with any prospects of play in the future; time goes so slowly with children.

This "deposition neurosis" is certainly one of the commonest forms of anxiety state in children. It can begin before the actual arrival of the second child.

D.C., a child of 3, was irritable and bad tempered. His mother, who was far gone in pregnancy, said she could do nothing with him, and he had always been so good. When I asked her if he knew what was happening, she said she felt he was too young to be told. I found that she had been in the habit of telling him stories on her knee for half an hour before his bath. Now that she had no knee, the ritual had been abandoned. I advised her to improvise. She should still give him his half hour with him close beside her and she should tell him why she could not nurse him any more. When I next saw her she said his old sunny disposition had returned.

When the new baby arrives, the older child reacts at first with interest. Wise parents see that he has his full share of attention. In those early days it is more often visitors than parents who do the damage. Whereas John was always a most important person he may be completely ignored in the rush to see the new baby. He is made to bathe in reflected glory, a process he doesn't always appreciate. "Aren't you a lucky boy to have such a dear little sister." It has been advocated that visitors should be warned against these dangers and they can actually increase the older child's pleasure and sense of responsibility by saying, "She is a lucky baby to have such a fine big brother to look after her".

Even without the interference of foolish visitors the first phase of interest soon passes, and the reactive stage sets in. Signs of acute jealousy may appear. The child shows by word or deed his disapproval of the new arrival. He may even seek to do physical violence to the baby or ask the mother to send her away. Jealousy may remain latent and parents will affirm he loves his little sister and is devoted to her, but anger and frustration must always be present. Until this small stranger arrived he had two parents to give him their undivided love and attention. Now at best, the love and attention must be divided and he has at most only half as much. He feels rather as we feel when we send off portions of our income to the Inspector of Taxes. What we feel is our own property is in fact taken from us against our wishes and we can do nothing about it, although we as adults can relieve our feelings by grumbling and putting the blame on the government, whereas the child is powerless to express his feelings direct. A show of jealousy meets with parental disapproval and so it readily goes underneath and becomes subconscious, giving rise when the strain is too great to symptoms of anxiety.

Intelligent parents, aware of the problem, do their best to prepare the older child beforehand, and to give him plenty of attention as he adjusts to the newcomer. The family settles down to the new routine and all appears to be going well, until suddenly and unexpectedly the older child becomes difficult when the baby is from nine months to a year old. There are two reasons for this; the parents may have been lulled into a sense of false security and relaxed their attention on the older child ; or the child may have realised that while the small baby helpless in her cot or pram was a poor rival, at a year when she is learning so many new tricks and is so very attractive, she has become a very real danger to his security. The jealousy reaction is not in fact confined to the first few weeks or months after the baby's birth but may be evident at any age in childhood.

T., aged 8, was brought to see me. Her mother was worried about her because she was always having nightmares and dreaming of fire. The house was burning or the bus was on fire or the car would catch alight. She also expressed a fear of her father. He might well fire the stairs at night and do her some mortal harm. The mother was an intelligent woman and co-operated well in treatment. T. had a young sister aged 6 who was as vivacious and pretty as T. was quiet and plain. The sister was recognised as "Daddy's girl". Three years prior to these attacks the young sister had had quite a severe hand burn. This injury had probably pleased T.; but of course the satisfaction was repressed because it gave rise to feelings of guilt. Both children were treated almost as twins. A point was reached when T's jealousy boiled over. She wished her sister burned again. The wish is repressed and in the dreams she is being burned often by her father, the hated rival's champion.

The mother was advised to pay T. very special attention and to devise some privileges for her to make her really superior instead of equal to her young sister. Riding lessons were given to T. and not to her sister who was "too young" to start. T. ceased having nightmares and her mother reported she was much happier in every way.

The normal child tends to live in the future, and not in the past. It is always, "when I am five—when I am big like Daddy, when it's my birthday, etc." The normal child wants to grow up and emulate and have the privileges of his parents. The arrival of a baby makes him stop and think. Instead of looking forward he tends to look backwards and remember with longing the joys of infantile dictatorship and importance. He may regress to infancy in bed wetting, thumb sucking and so on. Looking for this regression, I asked the mother of a small girl if the patient ever wet the bed. The mother said not and asked me why I had made the enquiry. When I explained she laughed and said, "Linda is always happy if she can be a baby. She likes to have her food pulped like baby's, and it is always bliss for her to be put into baby's cot".

Parents can readily appreciate this simple psychology and the remedy is equally simple; the older child must be compensated for being old. He must be made to realise that age has its privileges which are worth seeking.

I.W., aged 6, was a collier's son. His father brought him to see me because he was having such awful nightmares. He would awake screaming and see things in the bedroom. Trains would be bursting through the walls, and he was afraid to go up to bed or stay in the dark. He had a young sister aged nine months. When I asked about jealousy reactions, the father said he had noticed them. The boy would not allow the baby to touch any of his toys and was in many ways resentful. In a matter of 20 minutes during a busy surgery I explained the jealousy motive and the remedy.

I saw the father 3 months later and asked after his son. He beamed as he told me the nightmares had gone, and he had lost his fear of the dark and was much more friendly to his sister. He described the results as remarkable. When I asked what privileges he had given the boy, I must confess I felt they were equally remarkable. He was allowed to visit his grandmother half a mile away on his own ; he was given a few coppers to spend as he liked, to buy his own fish and chips and to visit the cinema alone (at 6!).

One is often amazed how receptive parents are to the psychiatric explanation of symptoms. I had to treat a small boy for several weeks for a serious diabetes mellitus. Soon after his recovery his older brother aged 12 came to see me with a bad knee for which I could find no explanation. I did discuss his brother with him ; but I had not made a psychiatric diagnosis on the knee. When I told his mother I had formed no definite opinion, she made the suggestion that perhaps the boy felt he should have some share of the attention that his brother had been earning. I think her diagnosis was correct.

Negativism is another symptom of the child's effort to maintain the parental attention, the goal of all small children. Anorexia and constipation are the commonest examples of this condition. Mothers of only children often fall victims to this ruse. Little Mary goes off her food. Special dishes are produced to please her and games are invented to coax the appetite. Each new idea of inducement and each fresh show of concern aggravates rather than improves the condition. It is usually quite difficult to treat the mothers of such children. They are so concerned about the child that they are convinced there is some organic cause for the poor appetite ; and as conscientious parents they are loath to admit that the trouble is the result of their own mismanagement and over concern. The proper lines to follow are as follows. Refusal of food is accepted without concern or dismay and no other food is proffered until the next meal. Eating between meals, sweets and so on are forbidden. When a clean plate is produced by the child, he must be congratulated and rewarded. The child soon learns he gets more fuss and attention by eating than by fasting.

K.B. was brought to see me because of constipation. He never had his bowels moved without a purge while his older brother was held up as a model of regularity and virtue. The mother was genuinely concerned about the child and convinced there was some organic basis. Small regular doses of liquid paraffin were tried but they had no effect. After three short sessions I made a bargain with the mother. I suggested that on getting home she should tell K. she was not going to mention the pot to him again or remind him of his duties. If however he had a motion and showed it to her she would reward him. If he was not normal at the end of two weeks I promised her I would get a second opinion. This latter was never necessary because the child became regular at once. He was only difficult because of his mother's ritual fuss over his habits.

The second infantile delusion could be described as the Divinity of Parents. To small children parents seem to be all good, all powerful, and all knowing. Only children are naughty, and while bad men are known to exist and may be read about in stories, like lions and robbers, the child does not expect to meet them in everyday life. Parents are immensely strong and immensely rich. While the child has to be content with a sixpence or a few coppers; the parent always has a pocket full of silver and a few bank notes as well. Parents are all knowing to a small child, because they always have an answer for any question the child may ask. The first infantile delusion disappears as soon as a new sibling is born or when the child goes to school. The second delusion fades out somewhere between the years 8–12. The child learns that parents are not completely honest and logical. Unfulfilled promises rankle, small deceptions are spotted and, perhaps most of all, incidents which savour of unfairness make a deep impression. One adult patient remembered vividly as a child arguing with his mother, who was a very religious woman, in an effort to evade a beating. "It says in the Bible you should forgive until 70 times seven". When his theology did not save him, his feelings were, "These people say one thing but do another. They tell you to believe the Bible but they do not obey it themselves".

Parents' knowledge is limited and as schooling advances, the child finds he knows things which the parent does not, or has forgotten. He also realises that the parents are not millionaires who can satisfy his every whim and fancy as they used to in infancy.

The purpose of the delusion is to give the small child a sense of security. How can harm come to him, when he is protected by two such omnipotent creatures?

Mrs. H. came to see me because M. aged 4 had developed an acute insomnia. She was put to bed at 7 o'clock but by 10–11 o'clock she was still wide awake. I had seen Mrs. H. in an anxiety state herself so that she knew something about psychotherapy. I told her that something was worrying M. and it was up to her to find out the problem. This she had to do by paying special attention to the child, and trying to get her confidence. Two weeks later Mrs. H. returned triumphant. She had solved the problem, and what was more important M. was behaving normally again.

She discovered that the girl's cousins across the street, whose parents were divorced, had told M. it was only a matter of time before her parents broke up the home. As soon as Mrs. H. had discovered the worry, both she and her husband reassured the child, and she started to sleep normally again.

When the child is deposed from the throne of babyhood by the arrival of a new baby, he still has his divine parents to protect and succour him. If these ideals are rudely shattered in infancy, the child develops a state of insecurity and becomes anxious. This happens if there is quarrelling between the parents or open vice such as drunkenness. In a quarrel both parents cannot be right, so that if one is right the other must be wrong and naughty. A friend of mine told me how on one occasion he and his wife were having a heated discussion on some matter. There was no question of a quarrel, it was just an argument. One of the children burst into tears and pleaded with them to stop fighting. To the child even a lively debate can appear like a quarrel. Insecurity is brought about when poverty makes the child realise there is really no food in the larder and no money in mother's purse for it. Anxiety can also come from reflected anxiety because it casts doubt upon this supposed perfection of the parents.

I was called in to see a small girl of 4 who had become manneristic and fearful of the dark. I asked the mother to come and see me at the surgery by herself. There I learned that the child had told her she still loved her Daddy, but she wasn't sure about her mother. The mother admitted she was very moody and the parent's irritability and the uncertainty of her temper was worrying the child. The mother was in fact suffering from effort syndrome. This was cleared in 3 sessions and before she had finished coming to see me she said the child too had quite recovered. The uncertain mood and temper of the mother had shaken the child's feelings of security. She was no longer certain of her mother's love. As soon as the mother became more confident in herself, more even in her mood, the child's anxiety abated too.

I saw a small boy of $2\frac{1}{2}$ with a bead in his nose. I tried unsuccessfully to remove it, and I had to refer him to hospital. I called to see him the next day. The bead had been pushed back into the naso pharynx and was swallowed. The child had quite recovered but was stammering badly. I asked if he had talked about doctors and hospitals since his experience, but the parents had avoided the subject. I told them to tell him how sorry they were that he had had to go to the doctor, and how painful his experiences must have been. The bead had to be removed, and such a thing would never happen again if he avoided pushing things up his nose. Two days later his stammer had completely gone. Not only had this child had an unpleasant experience, but the parents had connived at his sufferings; they had even held him down. He needed reassurance that they were still responsible for him : that they still loved him and that his experience was not a punishment because he had angered them.

The idea of the divinity of parents should have faded by the age of twelve or so. Some adults still have queer ideas about the perfection of their elders because they have never shed the delusion of the divinity of their parents. Such people are as liable as children to exhibit symptoms of anxiety when something happens that shakes their belief.

Mrs. M.S., a woman of 35, came to see me in an anxiety state of the depressive type which she had endured for two years. She was the only girl of the family and had four brothers. Her parents were very decent religious folk and she had a good upbringing. She married and had two children of her own. While her husband was away at the war her neighbours—an elderly couple, befriended her ; and this pair were identified with her parents, and became parent substitutes.

After the war her husband came home, and money began to disappear from the house. The young couple could not explain it ; each thought the other was careless. Then one day my patient remembered that when some money was lost, the neighbour's daughter, a woman of 26, had been in the house, and my patient had heard her open the desk as she came downstairs. They had lost a good deal of money from time to time and they reported their suspicions to the police.

The police were very pleased to get the report as the culprit had been suspect in many other petty thefts. My patient was upset when she found proceedings had been started and tried to withdraw the charge. The police would not agree and the case went forward to a conviction.

The old people next door turned on the younger couple in their anger over the shame that their daughter had brought on the family. They behaved with such cruelty and unfairness that life became almost unbearable. My patient admitted that she felt she could never trust anyone again. It took some five sessions of psychotherapy to get things sorted out, but she improved in health out of all recognition and has remained well ever since, although the neighbour's attitude which caused the depression remained unchanged. Her neurosis was due to the violent breaking up of the parent ideal, an infantile delusion which should have gone by puberty.

It thus behoves us as parents not to try and uphold the idea of parental perfection too long. The Victorian parent, as depicted in "The Barretts of Wimpole Street", was a tyrant, whose word was law, and whose utterances were not to be questioned. Such an attitude is obviously very wrong. There is no such thing as the perfect mother or father. The thoughtful parent will from time to time find he is wrong, and he should admit it to the child. Children have a great sense of fairness. The admission of an error, far from making the parent lose face, makes him a good sport. As parents we must see that our importance does not outlive its usefulness. In some ways disillusionment is to our own advantage. If we retain some regrets when our children discover that our goodness is not impeccable or our wisdom absolute, at least we are compensated when they grasp the fact that our wealth is not limitless, and that we have no fairy wand with which to satisfy their slightest whim.

The third delusion of childhood is the legend of immortality. The small child has no real conception of time. If he is told it is Christmas next week, that conveys the idea of some time in the future, a week, a month or tomorrow, it makes no difference. Christmas is just "coming". His three score years and ten expectation of life go far beyond anything he would possibly comprehend and stretch away into a future infinity. Children understand what is meant by death, and hardly need to have it explained. "That cat is dead" a small girl will say cheerfully to her younger sister. "You see it cannot move and it is all stiff". With such an immense span of life stretching before them, they feel that they themselves are immortal, and so are their immediate associates, brothers, sisters and parents. If a parent or a sibling dies, then the whole fantasy is shown to be false. The rude shattering of any infantile delusion renders the child anxiety prone, or it actually precipitates an anxiety state. In a case of serious illness, as long as the delusion holds, and the parents manage to maintain an atmosphere of calm security, the illness itself does not worry the small child. He still feels secure. But if the parents show great anxiety, the child is upset by the parents' agitation. In other words he is infected by parental anxiety, in much the same way as we see it in young animals. A clutch of partridge chicks who have never seen a human being show no signs of fear, but as soon as the mother bird spots the intruder and utters her warning cry, the nestlings go into a panic.

That a child can have a very real fear of death is illustrated in the following case.

L.S. was a man of 28 who was admitted to the neuro-psychiatric centre on the verge of delirium tremens. He had in fact a severe effort syndrome and could not or dare not go to sleep at night unless he had been well fortified by drink. He felt that one day he would drop dead. He blamed his heart which he was sure was affected.

He first became worried about his heart when putting up a tent. His heart started palpitating and he felt in a state of terror. He had had previous attacks of panic, the first occurring at the age of 6. He was playing with some hairy caterpillars which had barbed fur, and contact with them is liable to cause a rash. His mother saw him and told him to put them away as they were poisonous. For a while he obeyed her, but the discovery of more caterpillars started a new game. His mother found him, and told him "I have warned you. You will die now". His hands were tingling and he ran to her and asked her to wash them for him. She replied that it was too late. He could remember running in a panic to the stream, lying on his stomach and trying to wash his hands clean. He was terrified as he lay there waiting to die.

In actual fact his terror and insecurity had two roots. His mother's cruel threat had broken for him the myth of immortality. When he did not die he realised his mother was a liar and not the divine protector. In one fell blow two infantile fantasies were shattered. That his reactions were not just pure fear is shown by another experience he had at an even earlier age. He was playing by a stream when a snake approached him. He ran in terror to the house screaming for his mother, only to find the door locked. He had to race round to the back before he got inside to safety. When I asked him if he felt as bad on both occasions, he replied that the snake episode was not too bad, as he still had his mother to help him.

This legend of immortality is the last delusion to go. The mature adult should have a philosophic attitude towards death. Those who have been frightened by it, or have been brought face to face with it at an early age are rendered anxiety prone. Such sensitivity rarely leads to childhood neurosis, but those who are sensitive are candidates for effort syndrome and the like in later life. This delusion should be shed from seventeen to twenty-one, but many adults remain immature in this respect.

As in adult neuroses there are short cases. If some psychic trauma can be located which has occurred recently, trauma which accounts for the symptoms, it is usually easy to deal with.

A small girl of three started having nightmares. She could never remember what had frightened her in the morning. In looking for a cause of the trouble, the parents remembered that on the day prior to the first attack, she had fallen off a log into a deep pool and had to be pulled out. The parents tried to laugh off the incident, by saying how well she swam, and asking if she had seen any mermaids. The child accepted this phantasy and told neighbours of her adventure in these false terms. The fear and panic memories were repressed, only to emerge as nightmares. The parents were advised to remind her of the accident, and to rub in how unpleasant it had been for her. When they adopted this attitude the nightmares ceased promptly. That was seven years ago and bad dreams have never recurred.

If no obvious trauma can be seen in the environment of home or school, then one must analyse the situation in terms of the three infantile delusions. Has the child been deposed ; have the parents upset his faith in them ; or has illness or death in the family upset his sense of security. It is nearly always possible to discover some source of anxiety and if this is righted, recovery sets in. If a blank is drawn in every direction or no satisfactory response is obtained, then the services of a psychiatrist or a school psychologist should be secured.

What has been said so far applies largely to behaviour disorders. Psychomotor neuroses such as eneuresis, stammering and habit spasm are manifestations of a more profound disorder and are thus more difficult to tackle. Eneuresis has already been dealt with. Very few cases of stammering seem to appear in a general practitioner's surgery and those that do are better passed on to a speech clinic or a psychiatrist. Habit spasm or tic is worth tackling along general lines but it usually takes a long time to eradicate. The parents must be reassured that the habit is harmless and will pass. The less attention which is paid to it the better. Every effort must be made to discover a cause, and that dealt with in the usual way. Habit spasm is often symbolic and in itself often gives a pointer to the real trouble.

P.H. was a nervous youth of 15. He was the youngest of three brothers and his mother's favourite. He had a shrugging of his right shoulder which he was unable to control. At 11 he had a head shaking habit. These tics were both accounted for by severe emotional crises. The head shaking came on after he had been caned in front of his class at school for something he had never done. The significance of the shake was obvious. The shrugging of his right shoulder came on at 13 after a very tragic incident. His mother was a heart invalid. On one occasion the family went for a drive in the car and he sat in the back with his mother. She became ill and collapsed on to his right shoulder. She actually died before they reached home. Again the movement of the right shoulder clearly had significance. Discussion of these painful situations relieved anxiety and the habit spasm gradually faded out, but there was no dramatic improvement.

Before leaving the subject of psychiatry in childhood, I feel I should mention one of the awkward ages of childhood. At some time between the ages of 2 and 5, the child turns from the helpless infant who is rather plastic and suggestable into the more mature individual who has a mind and a will of his own. This metamorphosis may be a very unpleasant experience for the parents, as the child, who had previously been good and biddable, becomes definitely the reverse, bad and unruly. He wants this or that and, no matter how absurd the request, if it is not granted at once there is a scene. This "I want" phase usually lasts for a few months. Parents sometimes blame the child's nerves, and naturally any occasion for anxiety aggravates the condition. It is, however, in itself a perfectly natural phase as the passive infant discovers its own will and experiments with its actions on other people. The only essential treatment is to reassure the parents and tell them the phase will pass over. The child needs firm but very gentle treatment ; giving way will spoil it, but the ultra firm line might break it. The happy mean is needed. The child will quickly accept the value which it finds its parents ready to accord to its individual will. If they give way it will become and remain domineering: if they are too hard it will accept its weakness and remain weak and easily led all its life. If they can teach it to expect, and to give, fair treatment in comparison with other members of the family, it will grow up to be a fair minded and useful citizen.

Childhood ends at puberty, and with the physical change come certain changes in the psychological make-up. Psychoses in childhood are excessively rare, but at puberty schizophrenia can occur. In my experience anxiety states are rare at this stage, but this may be because the child at puberty keeps himself to himself and thus the anxiety passes unnoticed.

When all patients seen suffering from all forms of psychiatric illness aged 21 and under are grouped in age order, it can be seen that the incidence is lowest at 13, 14 and 15 (see p. 138).

At no age is the individual more aggressively withdrawn than at puberty. Reticence is not the hall mark of all adolescents, but the introverted quiet and solitary types become withdrawn and schizoid. If at this age an anxiety state arises, the patient is often unapproachable. He resents the intrusion of a doctor or a psychiatrist into his affairs.

Mrs. M. came to see me about D. age 14, because both she and her husband were worried about him. He kept talking to himself. He liked to be alone and would be found muttering to himself. He was excessively religious, and if they did not keep an eye on him he would pray for hours in the night. He was slow in doing things and had to be pushed along. He had changed from a jolly lad full of fun and jokes to a serious solitary mystic.

I thought at once of schizophrenia. Only one thing in his history made me question the diagnosis, and that was that his parents insisted that his school reports were good. I wrote to his school master who confirmed this, although he admitted his behaviour was strange. I sent him to see a psychiatrist who suggested it was an anxiety state of puberty. As things remained static for some months I sent him to see yet another psychiatrist who again suggested it was an

Age Incidence of Neuroses in Childhood

Age	No. of patients	3 Yearly Groups	
1	1		
2	9	1–3	16
3	6		
4	9		
5	9	4–6	27
6	9		
7	3		
8	5	7–9	13
9	5		
10	6		
11	1	10–12	12
12	5		
13	3		
14	3	13–15	8
15	2		
16	8		
17	8	16–18	31
18	15		
19	6		
20	16	19–21	37
21	15		

anxiety state. Time eventually confirmed the diagnosis though recovery was slow. The boy is now 16 and almost recovered. He is at work and doing well. There is no evidence whatsoever of schizophrenic deterioration.

The boy was psychiatrically unapproachable. He made me feel a complete worm for daring to intrude into his life, and I was impotent to help him directly. The local parson was a useful ally here. The boy was religious and had a great respect for the clergyman. I discussed the case with him, and the rapport the patient had with his minister helped him along.

The basis of such an anxiety state is probably a feeling of guilt over the problem of masturbation. One can never find out for certain because the patient will not co-operate.

Most behaviour problems in childhood yield readily to a simple form of therapy which is within the scope of the general practitioner. If neglected, the consequences of childhood anxiety may be far reaching and permanent. In view of this it would seem reasonable that such cases should be given radical treatment, and if this fails, specialist help should be sought. The mental health of children is quite as important as their physical well being. Happily, in this sphere of work the general practitioner is not working alone. He has a useful ally in the school psychologist who shares the burden of this great responsibility. Where such a friend is available, every opportunity should be made to make use of his services.

CHAPTER VIII

PSYCHIATRIC CONDITIONS IN THE AGED

AGED people are susceptible to all forms of psychiatric illness. In the last decade of life senile dementia is common, and the individual becomes a helpless empty shadow of himself. "Last scene of all that ends this strange eventful history, is second childishness and mere oblivion, sans teeth, sans eyes, sans taste, sans everything." Nothing can be done for these unfortunate people who become a great burden on their families. It is the relations who need the encouragement to persevere in their attentions. Besides dementia, the aged suffer from anxiety states, psychoses of all kinds, and transient symptoms of mental illness such as delusions, hallucinations and paranoid ideas. Old people who are physically ill often have transitory mental symptoms which clear as health improves, and are of as little consequence therefore as the confusion and mild delirium of a child with fever.

While the psychiatric diseases from which the aged suffer are the same, the treatment is of necessity rather different from that suitable for younger patients. Anxiety states for example can be treated only most superficially by psychotherapy. The mind of an old person is too rigid to accept any psychological explanation of his symptoms. Just as the circumstances promoting anxiety in childhood have to be smoothed out as far as possible, so for the aged the environment must usually be changed to suit the patient. It is not possible to make an old person adapt himself to conditions which upset him.

Anxiety States

It is not surprising that anxiety states should be quite common in old people. There are many new and potent stresses and strains imposed on an individual as old age approaches. By far the commonest difficulty to be faced is the conscious waning of physical powers, the inability to participate in the activities which the patient has enjoyed as long as he can remember. Hand in hand with the irritation of physical failure is the fear of becoming dependent, the fear of what will happen when they are no longer able to look after themselves. Many old people who have, with stout hearts, remained proud and independent all their lives, dread this stage more than death itself. The fact that today the welfare state has removed the fear of destitution and of the workhouse, has doubtless relieved some of the anxieties of the aged, but it cannot alter the fact that in extreme age or in sickness the old person must still become dependent on other people to look after him. Fifty years ago people insured against this difficulty by having large families. Among the working classes it was by no means always lust which made a hasty marriage necessary—it was policy to be sure that a man's mate was fertile before taking her as a permanent partner. The era of large families has gone ; with fewer children, and each of them anxious for a higher standard of living, the burden of the aged falls more heavily on each. Thus, the problem facing the aged will become even more difficult in the future.

The old person knows he is nearing the end of the road, and symptoms of physical illness may be viewed with considerable apprehension as the beginning of the end. Some, especially those who have had neuroses before, make themselves miserable with anticipation and graft an anxiety state on to every physical ailment that they contract, though the vast majority of old people bear physical infirmity with fortitude and remain hopeful to the end.

The treatment of anxiety states in the aged must be modified to meet the peculiar circumstances and problems from which they arise. The various lines of approach possible are as follows:

(a) Reassurance

When one performs a complete physical examination on a young person, one can usually exclude physical disease with a fair degree of accuracy. In the aged it is not so easy. The heart may appear normal in every way and there may be no evidence of any physical disease, and yet the patient may die of a coronary occlusion or a stroke a few hours after such a negative examination. At the same time if one senses that the symptoms of the old person are largely functional and there is no evidence of organic disease, one must take a risk and state that for his or her age the patient is perfect. Nature does help us in senility. I have several old people with incipient heart failure, but they live quite comfortably because their level of activity is so low, it throws no great strain on the diseased organ.

Mrs. M.G., aged 79, sent for me because she had had an attack of acute epigastric pain. There was no evidence of gross organic disease and I suspected a cholecystitis, a diagnosis I had no reason to question until I was present on the third occasion and found she was suffering from paroxysmal auricular fibrillation which produced pain from cardiac ischæmia. Digitalis has almost cut out the attacks, which when they do occur are relieved by liberal doses of pethidine. Five years have passed and she is still alive, and happy because she is well cared for by her family. Her activity is minimal.

This case illustrates the risks we are bound to run in reassuring the aged. When I first examined her I found no evidence of heart disease, in fact I reassured her that her heart was normal for her age. The risk of being proved wrong is one which I feel must be taken unless old people are to be plunged into a state of anxiety by carefully worded non-committal remarks. Once I had discovered her heart was at fault I told her what was happening in words she could understand. The case also illustrates how by a general lowering of vitality, old age reduces the importance of certain physical disabilities ; disabilities which would be seriously crippling in the young and vigorous. The old woman has been able to enjoy five years of senescence with a heart capable of very little effort.

With young neurotics, the physical examination is once and

for all. This is not so with the aged. A periodic examination is necessary in old people both to keep a check on one's diagnosis, and to reassure the patient. Reassurance is greatly enhanced by a periodic check up. It is only natural that they should feel that the passage of time, a few months or a year, should possibly be accompanied by some change in their general physical well being. Thus it is that the aged diabetic is often more interested in the state of his pulse than his urine. Thus, too, it is that we find healthy but old people periodically attending the surgery with a comparatively small symptom and a great deal of anxiety. If they are examined thoroughly and reassured that their general condition is still quite satisfactory, the presenting symptom is quickly forgotten. The symptom was important only as a possible red light warning them of impending general dissolution.

Mrs. B.S., aged 75, comes to see me annually. She first came three years ago convinced there was something growing in her throat. There was no evidence of organic disease apart from hypertension. She was reassured that there was no physical cause for her trouble, and it was a common symptom of nerves in women. I saw her regularly for a month and the trouble faded away. A year later she came with a bad head. Again a complete examination was made with the same results. She thought she had blood pressure. I told her this was so, but it did not cause her headache and that the level of her hypertension was no cause for alarm. She came back once more after an interval of about a year. She had a persistent cough. This I thought might be due to incipient left heart failure, but a physician found no evidence of heart failure on investigation. The cough disappeared and once more she is reassured and feeling well until some new symptom arises. The disappearance of the old symptoms is a great help in reassuring her about new ones.

(b) Occupational Therapy

The second weapon of psychotherapy is to encourage every possible interest. The old lady must be encouraged to do all kinds of work within her power. It may be dusting or washing up, or merely arm chair jobs such as darning socks. The old man must be encouraged to potter about in his garden, gather sticks for the winter or glean a basket of coal off the road-side. If all activity must temporarily be suspended, the hope of future activity must be encouraged. The winter is easier to endure if the old man feels that when the spring comes he will be able once more to sow a few seeds in his garden. Those who can read are indeed fortunate. Mental activity certainly delays the onset of senescence. The man who can enjoy a good book can bear his infirmities better than his brother who is no reader. The wireless, and to-day television, both help to entertain the aged and keep them in touch with events. Unfortunately few old people take kindly to the radio and may complain they cannot stand the noise. Perhaps it is too late to become a radio fan when one is a septuagenarian, although I know at least one old lady who did not have a wireless in her house until she was 74 and has since become an addict.

It is unfortunate too that the radio is so rarely used as effectively as it might be. Of the old people who listen, few do so regularly or have their favourite programmes which they can anticipate with pleasure. The most fortunate old people are those who remain active church members. Religion not only proffers some hope for the future, but with an active parish priest the aged are still members of a society which takes a real interest in them.

Independence should be preserved as long as possible. All too often children persuade the old person to give up his home to live with them. After a few months the old person is a burden to the younger family, and he is depressed by feeling he is an unwanted intruder. It is often necessary and desirable for children to care for aged parents but it is no easy solution and independence should be encouraged for as long as possible. With solitary old folk there is the risk that they may die suddenly alone and unattended, but in such independent spirits it is a risk worth taking, when weighed against the miseries of premature dependence and the irritations of an unhappy home life. The old person who feels inadequate because of his failing powers, must be made to feel he is still of importance to his family circle. So often he feels he is a burden when such is not the case. In old age an old man becomes a figure head like the king. Our soveriegn does no actual ruling, but he is a vital figure head in our society. It is the same with the head of the family. Even if he does nothing, he is an honoured figure head and there is no need to vindicate his position.

(c) Moulding Circumstances

As has already been stated, circumstances must as far as possible be smoothed out for the aged. It is not possible for them to make much in the way of adaptation. Like children they must be assured of a fair share of family affection, and this is not always easy. Children are essentially lovable, whereas the aged can be most difficult and trying. This only underlines the desirability of encouraging old people to live on their own as long as possible. Distance does make the heart grow fonder. Visits from children and grandchildren are a real joy, whereas living with the family may be over-whelming. Grandchildren are best prescribed in small and frequent doses.

It is wrong to try and regiment the aged. They need more than their fair share of their own way. For this reason physical treatments and routines need not be too zealously applied. The aged diabetic finds great difficulty in adapting herself to the new regime. A strict diet is no more important than her peace of mind. If an occasional cake will please her without danger, it should be allowed. Happiness is more important than a normal sugar content in the blood.

Psychoses

One of the commonest psychiatric illnesses in the aged is that of depression. It is almost impossible to differentiate the reactive type from a true endogenous depression. Fortunately differentiation is unnecessary as the treatment is the same in any case. Insomnia is usually an outstanding symptom, and often if this alone is dealt with, the patient improves. The depression may often simulate organic disease like a depressive graft. This was illustrated in Case T.S. already described in Chapter V and also in the following cases:

Mrs. H.I., aged 85, was under my care for diabetes, discovered a couple of months previously. She became very depressed and started waking at nights, bathed in perspiration which was so heavy that she had to be changed twice or thrice during the night. The symptoms suggested hyper insulin attacks and the evening dose of insulin was stopped, but it had no effect on the sweats. A thermometer was left with her daughter and there was never any evidence of a fever. She became worn out and miserable and would readily burst into tears. She did not respond well to barbiturates, but chloral hydrate (gr. 30) at night, made her sleep well and both the sweating and the depression left her.

Mrs. F.C.C., aged 86, had a cough and fever bouts at night. One of my colleagues was treating her, and she became so ill that he decided she had a low grade pneumonia and so put her on to sulphonamides. I saw her after she had been ill for a week. I knew her very well and was impressed by the misery written on her face, which was usually so cheerful. I found no gross evidence of organic disease, but she had had almost complete insomnia for 10 days. The hot bouts she complained of came on at night and distressed her greatly. Both she and her family felt she was about to die. I was called out at 2.0 a.m. to witness an attack on one occasion. There was no temperature and her pulse was steady and slow. She responded well to sodium amytal gr.iii and with this dosage the attacks ceased and she slept well. After 4 good nights I told her she could get up and she progressed rapidly, once the sleep rhythm had been re-established.

Death comes to most people stealthily, "as a thief in the night". If death is in any way anticipated, it is usually a symptom of depression.

All aged anxiety states and depressions do not respond so happily, and many of the most trying and time consuming cases in the practice are those which have become chronic and are indeed confirmed hypochondriacs.

Transient hallucinations are not infrequent in the aged who are toxic. One, a woman of 73, used to have the most vivid and pleasant visions of crowds around her smiling and waving to her. She had no insight into her condition and indeed much enjoyed the spectacle. She was suffering from heart failure ; and as her condition improved her visitors left her, and insight returned. "It wasn't right to see such things, was it?" she asked me on one occasion. Relatives are often worried by such symptoms ; but if they do occur in relation to organic disease they are usually transient.

If they occur insidiously in one physically fit, the prognosis is not so good. However they may cause a little trouble unless they are accompanied by paranoid ideas.

Mrs. S.E.H., aged 86, was quite convinced her husband aged 90 was having an affair with the milk girl. The delusion was quite fixed and to some extent systematised. She used to tell her mirror image all her troubles and when her husband, in a misguided attempt to reassure her of his affection, put his arm on her shoulder, she said at once, "There you go again fondling the woman—and you do look soft". This condition has been going on for two years and the patient is very difficult, as like all paranoid people she feels everyone is in league against her. She is fortunate in that she has plenty of children to look after her and to bear with her peculiarities.

Delusions usually worry the relations far more than the patient. Mrs. I.H., aged 84, had a very bad memory and her mind wandered a good deal. She would forget her living family and enquire after her father. She would make absurd suggestions about visiting friends long dead. She was lucid at times and just as strange a few hours later. She was looked after by a very capable daughter, but life became very difficult for both, as the daughter would insist on trying to correct the old lady's delusions. I talked to the patient and she rather reluctantly admitted that at times she did get mixed up. I told her this was very common among old people and nothing to worry about, but that she must be guided by her daughter who had a younger and better memory. I advised the daughter to ignore the delusions as far as possible. If the mother was difficult, this should be explained to her when she was lucid and more co-operative. This compromise made life much easier for both parties. Many people do not realise that you cannot argue a patient out of a delusion.

As in the younger age groups, gross hysteria may be a prelude to a more serious illness.

J.B., aged 63, was brought out of the pit in a state of collapse. Physical examination revealed no abnormality : but he was very enfeebled and weak. He lost his memory and became very deteriorated with incontinence of urine and fæces. He was sent to a mental hospital where presenile psychosis was diagnosed. He did not like the experience, and rapidly improved. He was sent home after a month and has remained fairly well for the past 2 years. He has a hopeless memory and is incapable of doing much in the house or garden, but he can look after himself and is socially well. The sudden weakness and deterioration was a hysterical overlay on a slowly progressive presenile dementia.

Aged folk should only be certified as insane in the last resort. Active treatment is unlikely to be available and they often curl up and die when removed from their own fireside, and everyone feels a sense of remorse when this happens. The relatives are inclined to think the patient has been neglected and should never have been allowed to go to a hospital. Elderly patients are not very welcome at mental institutions as they occupy useful beds which might be better employed. Every infirmary for the aged should have a ward for the mentally sick, so that those who have the misfortune to end their latter days hopelessly insane can avoid the stigma of a mental hospital. They don't need much restraint as they are physically incapable because of their age. It is conceivable that an old person might have to be transferred from the old age infirmary to a mental hospital, but such an event would be rare ; and it is very much easier for all concerned to have a stepping stone, thereby excusing the family direct responsibility for sending an aged parent to a mental institution.

CHAPTER IX

HYSTERICAL REACTIONS

It has been shown that the psychiatric case most commonly seen in general practice is that of the patient with an anxiety state. This condition recovers with treatment in a few weeks. The melancholic has to be sustained through his sufferings for a longer period, but the condition is usually self limiting and the patient eventually recovers. The hysteric is a kind of psychiatric jack-in-a-box. Treatment may relieve his symptoms for a time, but sooner or later, they pop up again, often in some new guise. A man is treated for urinary symptoms and his troubles clear. Three months later his bladder is causing no trouble but he is having blackouts. The hysteric is not necessarily a chronic attender at the surgery. He recovers, but never for very long. He is bowled over again more readily than the normal individual. One can expect him to appear for his sick notes once or twice a year; and once "on the club", he is reluctant to be signed off, though loud in his protests of his eagerness to work and his dislike of troubling the doctor. Often considerable powers of persuasion are necessary to get him back to work. Treatment may relieve symptoms, but it is beyond the powers of the general practitioner to cure or change the hysteric.

Textbook definitions of hysteria are varied and most confusing. Ross (i) describes it as "when a patient answers difficulties with a negative response". Kraines (ii) defines it as "a symptom complex presumably characterised by any change of function which is not on an organic basis". Every textbook referred to devotes a long paragraph to the definition, and at the end one is left with the feeling that hysteria is just another functional illness. It is indeed difficult to give a pithy definition. Barbour's description (iii) is to my mind the most apt. "It is a form of behaviour, rather than a specific illness". The anxiety state has been defined as a reaction to stress and strain. The hysterical reaction has the same motivation, but the individual is emotionally and socially either immature or stunted.

Hysterical Personality and Behaviour

The hysteric is usually, although not always, a person of subnormal intelligence. His characteristics come under three main headings, namely egocentricity, suggestability and lack of insight. They are all typical of a childish immature personality.

Egocentricity

In the hysteric the first delusion of childhood has never really faded out. He is selfish and eager to hold the centre of the stage. He is often ambitious but he is inefficient and has poor staying power. He is emotionally immature. If a show of rage will not achieve his object he becomes a pathetic object of tears. He will do silly things to impress. The hysteric is the kind of person who makes headline news in certain daily papers, and inconveniences the whole community by disappearing dramatically for a few days after some trivial quarrel with his wife. He is ready to provoke a stir by threatening suicide and may even attempt to do it in a half hearted way. This desire for the limelight makes him histrionic and in illness his symptoms are often dramatic, such as a fit or collapse. He exaggerates his feelings or his activities to gain effect. If he admits to masturbation he does it seven times a day. If he claims to promiscuity it will be in a fantastic number of conquests. He is self centred and his affection for others is shallow. He is always wanting favours and is a master of flattery when he wants some privilege. In dealing with these people, it is as well to remember Ross's dictum (i) "Beware of the gratitude of the hysteric".

Suggestability

The second delusion of childhood, namely the omnipotence of parents, has also failed to disappear. Like a child the hysteric is suggestable, and too ready to believe what others tell him. Well meaning relatives by their sympathy and stories often suggest illnesses for him to copy. Their accounts often leave gaps which have to be filled in from his imagination and because his knowledge of anatomy is limited, his symptoms frequently differ characteristically from those of organic disease, as in glove and stocking anæsthesia. He is prone also to imitate others. He feels ill, and has a pain in his chest, when a neighbour has a heart attack. It is because of his increased suggestability that he is an easy subject for hypnosis. It is possible to use this in treatment but undesirable because many people are fearful of it, and in any case it is unnecessary. Just as friends and neighbours can suggest him into feeling ill, so the doctor with a good rapport can persuade him to feel well again.

Lack of Insight

This is a most significant factor in hysteria. The anxiety state is able to perceive how the stress and strain of environment can affect his feeling of well being, and almost from the start one can sense that the patient approves of the line of approach. The hysteric stands aloof. While he may appreciate intellectually that his symptoms started when some dramatic or unpleasant event took place, he cannot correlate the two events. This lack of insight produces the characteristic "belle indifference" of the hysteric. He can be strangely detached and calm over gross symptoms which would fill a normal person with horror, and views his paralytic arm with apparent unconcern.

Mrs. A. H. was a fat old woman of 70. She had incipient heart failure and lived most of her life in an armchair. She resented her restricted life and looked with envy at her husband who was small, thin and extremely active for his age. She complained bitterly about her invalidism and became extremely depressed. One day I was sent for in a hurry. She had gone blind. I found her in bed and surprisingly serene as she told me flatly that she could not see a thing. The blink reflex was present, the pupils reacted to light and the discs were normal. The family all felt she had had a stroke, and was about to die and were therefore agitated and distressed. She was calm and almost cheerful. Her depression and long string of complaints had gone. After a few days her vision slowly returned, and with it her depression. She had in fact for a few days exchanged hysterical blindness for her reactive depression, and while apparently blind she seemed unperturbed by the gravity of her symptom, and of course she had no insight into her condition.

In any psychological condition, be it a psychosis or a neurosis, roughly speaking the prognosis is good in proportion to the insight. In paranoia there is no insight and the prognosis is as bad as it can be. The typical anxiety state has insight, and therefore actively assists one in psychotherapy. The hysteric who is deficient in insight has to be wooed away from his symptoms, which is often a very tiring and time consuming business. Again, it should be noted that even if one actually removes the symptoms, the basic hysterical personality remains unchanged.

Thus the hysteric may be defined as an emotionally immature individual, who produces a symptom complex of a functional nature, and who is incapable of correlating his symptoms with circumstances.

Clinically there are two distinct types of this condition, namely, frank hysteria, with its histrionic manifestations, and hystero-anxiety.

Frank Hysteria

This consists of such dramatic manifestations as the fugue, the fit, paralysis, blindness and so on. They are symptoms which never occur in a normal individual and the condition is usually fairly easy to diagnose, but it is comparatively rare.

M.H., a small girl aged nine, was brought to see me with a wry neck. Her story was that in class a boy behind her put something round her neck and pulled it tight. This had, of course, "injured" her neck. The teacher noticing the commotion called the child to the front of the class and was very angry. The wry neck was however an excellent defence mechanism. She kept it up all day and in the end she was told to see a doctor. Her mother brought her up the next morning. I laid her on my couch and persuaded her to tell me the story, with her feelings towards the boy who had hurt her, the teacher and the school in general. All the time I was straightening her neck and encouraging her by saying how well she was doing. In five minutes the spasm had gone and her neck was straight, much to her mother's delight. Parent and child went home far more contented than I was myself. To my mind little had been gained by the removal of the symptom, as neither the child nor her mother appeared to have any appreciation of why the symptom had developed. However that was three years ago and there has been no recurrence.

Mr. W.G., aged 29, came to see me very worried about himself. He had been kicked on the head while playing football and had had a blackout lasting for several hours. He could remember asking his way to the football ground and the next thing he remembered was waking up in hospital. The windows were closed and he thought at once he was in a mental hospital. Since his discharge from hospital things had begun to seem unreal to him. When watching people doing ordinary jobs, they seemed to be unreasonable about them. The houses in the village appeared to be different. Doors appeared where they were not before. The village had changed and changed for the worse. Trains passing half a mile away, seemed closer. Horse traffic seemed to fill the streets at night. He found himself questioning everything that happened and he added picturesquely, "life in general seems like a pantomime".

This man was an office worker with an intelligence above average. He was a small short sighted man who had married a very domineering young woman. She did not approve of his playing football. His attitude towards her was ambivalent, in that while he loved her as his wife, he resented her attitude to his interest in sport. On his way to play football his mind was divided. He wanted to play, but disliked his wife's disapproval. The amnesia was hysterical and not traumatic. The actual trauma was trivial, no one could say how he was hurt. The period of retrograde amnesia was too long for trauma, extending as it did from an hour or so before the accident. The whole incident offered an admirable escape mechanism from his difficulties. To stop playing football because of an injury was far more honourable than merely to satisfy the whims of an overbearing wife.

To get the full picture one has to go further back in his life. In the previous summer he had played cricket at the local mental hospital, where he had recognised a one time schoolmaster, who had gone insane because of a head injury. In spite of "being unconscious" he knew he had had a head injury and he knew, too, its ominous significance. Thus when he did come round he was "in a mental hospital" so he thought. He started worrying about his own sanity and his anxiety produced the queer ideas and methods of thought, just as heart worry produces cardiac symptoms.

I was at first uncertain of the diagnosis, but the possibility of hysteria was confirmed by a psychiatrist. After reassurance by the specialist he reported he was better and refused to have any further psychotherapy. This is the typical attitude of the hysteric. He has remained well over the past two years, but I was left with the feeling that he had very little interest or insight into his condition.

Hystero-Anxiety

This is merely an anxiety state in a hysterical personality. It is much more common than frank hysteria. The diagnosis is not obvious from the start. One is faced by an apparent anxiety state and it is only as psychotherapy progresses without achieving results that one realises the case is complicated by the hysterical personality with lack of insight. The symptoms are those of any anxiety state, and while one can perhaps persuade the patient into a better state of health, he does not have the appreciation of a normal anxiety state or the same satisfactory response to treatment.

J.H. was a man aged 33. While on holiday in Blackpool, something suddenly "went crack in his head", and he felt collapsed and ill. He was treated at Blackpool at first and I saw him two weeks after the incident. There were no signs of serious physical disease, but I felt the trouble might have been a sub-arachnoid hæmorrhage. He was referred to a neurologist who decided the case was functional. He failed to improve on simple reassurance, and so four months after the first attack I undertook psychotherapy.

He had many complaints. Pains reached from the back of his legs to his head. His legs went weak so that he could hardly move. He had churning feelings in his stomach. He had pains in his left ear which "hurt like a boil". Occasionally he had "comical feelings" during which he trembled all over !

This man, who had an average I.Q., was a taxi driver and was working up a flourishing business. He was very abstemious in his habits and had bought his own cottage and the one next door for his mother.

The basic trouble was not difficult to locate. His wife whose intelligence was probably subnormal, had had an affair with a builder who had been working on the premises. My patient had tricked them into an admission of guilt. For a time the couple lived apart, but as this was inconvenient for business purposes he took her back and decided to let bygones be bygones, but he continued to feel very sore about the whole matter and made little effort either to forgive or to forget what had happened.

In this humour he went for a holiday to Blackpool with his wife and there she unfortunately added insult to injury. They had gone to a café for a meal and while his wife sat at the table, he had ordered the food from the counter. On returning to his table, his wife, who had been forgiven so magnanimously, accused him of paying too much attention to the girl behind the counter. They quarrelled violently, he left the café boiling with wrath and indignation and when he got outside "his head went crack".

All the psychiatric evidence pointed to a psychological explanation of his feelings. This was supported by the reassurance of the neurologist and a psychiatrist. After five sessions with him he felt strong enough to start work again, but was far from well. I have had to see him periodically for the past year. He keeps at work and is in fact much better, but he just hasn't the mental capacity to correlate symptoms with events. Convincing evidence to corroborate my views was produced by free association (see Chapter III) but he just cannot mentally digest it. He is living on reassurance. He is reassuring himself by keeping at work and making a good living, and beyond re-enforcing and repeating reassurance to him, I have done little to help him. I have certainly achieved no radical reorientation of his attitude towards his symptoms.

Mrs. E.L., aged 28, came to see me complaining of claustrophobic symptoms. These were not serious but during the interview I discovered she was the child of a young woman who had been seduced by her uncle. Her mother had died at childbirth, and as a baby she had been adopted by a childless married aunt. What the patient really wanted was some reassurance about marriage. She was about to be wed and feeling she had poor inbred stock she wondered if she was right to marry and have children. I reassured her on these matters and gave her my usual premarital instructions.

She fell pregnant within four months of marriage and had a normal delivery of a perfectly normal little boy. She came up later for advice on contraception and I referred her to a neighbouring woman practitioner to be fitted with an occlusive pessary. However things went wrong and almost to the date she had a second child, a girl, a year after the first baby. The delivery was normal; but her convalescence was painfully slow. She had no energy and could not cope with her older child who was taken over by her foster mother. Physical examination revealed no cause for her state of inertia so psychotherapy was started.

As a child she had been strictly brought up by her foster mother, who dressed her like a doll and refused to let her mix with the village children. This attitude of superiority was quite inconsistent because any naughtiness was blamed on the lecherous uncle who had begotten her. She won a scholarship to a secondary school, and incredible as it sounds, she overheard the schoolmaster tell her mother a certain superior secondary school would never accept an illegitimate child. She was offered a second choice but she was so furious about it she refused to go at all. All these feelings of anger were kept to herself as she knew she could find sympathy from no one. She left school at 14 and then helped mother at home in an isolated country cottage. Life was dull and uninteresting. Her foster mother and father slept in different rooms and there was a very strained atmosphere in the house. She somehow learned that her grandfather had left her a legacy of £1000 to be used for her education. She saw a lawyer who agreed she could use it as she wished for educational purposes. She decided at 17 to leave home and take up shorthand and typing. There was great opposition to this from her foster mother, but she won her way through and went to college. There she did very well and on passing her exams she was taken on the staff of the college. Then began the happiest years of her life, working among people who respected her as the capable person she really was. The war came, and her sense of duty drove her into the land army. She served there for four years and she stuck it out although she hated the work. Neurosis at this stage would have made an easy escape ; but she never showed signs of any illness. After the war she returned to an office for a year, then married and became a farmer's wife in a lonely secluded farm. After the birth of her second child her neurosis came to a head. She had no energy, could not do her work, had terrible panic attacks when left on her own and generally felt very ill. I saw her in one panic attack. She was pale, and shaking from head to foot. Her condition was pitiable. She hated to be left alone ; but circumstances were such that she could not always have company.

Psychotherapy revealed great hatred against her foster mother, and after a few sessions she had worked everything out for herself. She said she knew she was not physically ill. She could in fact see an underlying purpose in her neurosis. She had concluded that her present illness was a protest against having her first child back from her mother. She wanted to have him back, but as soon as she felt well enough to do so, an attack came on and she had to put off the family reunion.

Here she had intellectual insight, and she had worked out the psychopathology for herself; but it did not relieve her symptoms. I felt she should be a good case because the way she had broken away from home, and served four years in the land army had demonstrated she had both intelligence and some fine character traits. I passed her on to a psychiatrist, as I felt I was not skilled enough to deal with her case. Unfortunately there was some mix up and she saw a junior consultant who advised her to go to a mental hospital for a time. That shattered her. She developed a strong negative transference against all doctors, and against me in particular. A hospital for neuroses was suggested and this was firmly turned down; and she has refused to see any doctor ever since. From her husband I have learned that it is now two years since she visited the village a mile away and her mother still has the older child. She has become a kind of hermit preferring to live with her symptoms rather than face an institution for a few months. Had her troubles been due entirely to anxiety, they should have cleared as she came to appreciate their origin. The persistence of symptoms indicated the presence of a hysterical element and a much more profound psychopathology.

These two cases illustrate the passive kind of hysteric who is willing to settle into a permanent state of complaining hypochondriasis and inactivity. There is another more active type who is equally prone to spells of illness. This active hysteric is so eager to hold the centre of the stage that he is often ambitious beyond his capacity. He aims at some impossible target and when he fails, he is prostrate with grief and annoyance. He can never see that he is in any way responsible for his failure. It is always ascribed to others or he claims to have had more than his share of bad luck. It is usually a waste of time to try to point out his share of responsibility in his misfortunes, but he should be encouraged to pour out his troubles. It can then be suggested that in spite of his bad luck he is still capable of doing some job of work. He should be loudly praised for any real achievement, and as far as possible guarded against over-reaching himself.

J.E. was a man of 30 who came to see me because he was run down. He was very worried about himself and full of symptoms. Physical examination was negative but his history was suggestive. Below average intelligence he was full of ambitions. He tried to do well at school but his master was very hard on him and "broke his spirit". Leaving school he went to a factory, but he did not enjoy the work which was too monotonous. At 18 he joined the Navy to "better himself". He had a cycle accident in which his face was badly cut up, and when he had recovered he was discharged from the service. He went to the brickyard but found the work hard and unattractive. While at this job he married, but his wife was prudish and frigid and refused to have intercourse with him. The war came along and he joined up and went abroad. In India he developed a severe hepatitis and kidney stones which kept him hospitalised for a considerable time. His wife stopped writing to him and he felt very wretched and ill. The matter was taken up with the Welfare Officer and soon after his demobilisation he was divorced. He was awaiting the absolute decree when he came to see me. I listened to his story, reassured him about his physical health and he went back to work in a factory. He remarried as soon as he could and after six months he came to see me in trouble again. He wanted a thorough examination as he thought he had venereal disease. His wife was expecting and he feared his child might be infected. There was no evidence of venereal disease and his W.R. was negative. He confided in me that his wife was a worry to him as she was dirty and careless in the home, very different from his mother. I interviewed his wife and she complained that he was always nagging her. He gave her a fair share of his earnings and in every other respect he was a good husband, but they did not appear to get on together as when they were first married. I saw him again and praised him for his wise handling of the family finances. I told him most couples had a difficult shake down period, and the pregnancy early in marriage tended to make it more difficult. I suggested if he praised his wife's good qualities rather than criticised her failures it would be better for both of them. It took me a month to persuade him that he could work in spite of his difficulties but once started I never saw him again for two years. On this last occasion he came down in a great state. He had pains in his neck and head, and felt he might collapse. He was sure he had blood pressure. I asked him how he was getting on and out came all his troubles. He had tried to better himself by working on the coal face, but after a week the manager had put him on a new job, with an inferior wage. When he asked why this had happened he was told he was not a suitable person for such work. I told him I thought the manager was right and that his present earnings of £9 a week were quite enough to keep him and his family. Life did not consist in earning big wages. Then he told me of a second disappointment. He was bent on taking a place in the ambulance team, but he always found himself the patient! I told him that as the patient he would learn a great deal from other people's mistakes. I suggested that while he was willing he did not learn easily but that in the end he could master first aid. "If you had asked me whether you should take your deputy's examination, I would say it was too hard for you, but you should manage your first aid." He then told me he had already sat for deputy, but had failed that too. His home life was now going well. He was a tryer and ambitious and I found plenty on which I could praise him. He said he felt much better for talking to me and could he come and see me again if he had any more difficulties. I have not seen him since, but I have no doubt that he will turn up again before long.

Many hysterics have a low I.Q. and their inferior intelligence renders them inadequate when the stress and strain of life becomes too great. They are quite incapable of accepting a psychiatric view of their illness, but even they can sometimes be persuaded back to work.

K.S., a woman of 40, had not worked for 10 years and was coming up month by month for her certificate labelled "Thyrotoxicosis". She was having no active treatment and there were no signs of the condition. I had her B.M.R. taken at the local hospital and it was normal. She lived a dull empty life with ageing parents. When I asked her why she did not work, she replied she was too ill to work. I gently but firmly told her the reverse was the case. She felt ill because she did not work. This old cliché is quite useful. "We only get out of life what we put into it." By winning her confidence and with persuasion I made her accept my idea, that once she was settled into a job she would feel better and not worse. After four months of patient prodding she took the plunge and worked steadily for two years. Then she had her teeth out and was off for four months. She went back for six months and is on my hands again at present.

J.K., a man aged 55, is a typical case. In his youth he fell astride the shaft of a cart and severely injured his testicles. He married but has had no children. He is on the state insurance for six to eight weeks every few months complaining of a lump in the throat and pains all over, due he believes to his accident. With encouragement and persuasion he eventually goes back to work for another 3 or 4 months.

Undoubtedly these low I.Q. hysterics are a great strain on one's patience and time, but by acting the part of father, mother and general adviser, one can get some work out of them, whereas if one takes the line of least resistance they would be complete parasites on society. There is little satisfaction in dealing with such cases but it is a social duty to try to help them. An average of six months' work per year is better than none at all.

In the army I had a young man of 19 under my care. His I.Q. was 96. His father was a senior government official and his two brothers were of university standard. This boy was the black sheep of the family because he was a misfit. When I asked him how many there were in the family he said four, and a moment later corrected himself. Clearly he wasn't really in the family. He was an outsider. This youth had the most spectacular attacks of hysteria. He would burst out crying and scream in his agitation, while nurses ran to comfort him and to keep him in bed. When I knew him really well he told me confidentially, he got great satisfaction from these attacks. As soon as there was a lull in the operations, an extra loud scream would result in renewed efforts on the part of the nurses. He had everyone completely at his beck and call and he consciously enjoyed it although he did not consciously initiate the attacks. The conscious production of symptoms is malingering. This boy was a typical hysteric not far removed from the malingerer. The psycho-pathology of his attacks was simple. He was being forced beyond his intellectual pace ; he could not gain the affection and respect of his parents by his achievements in life but found he could get plenty of attention by throwing one of his attacks. It was easy to establish a good rapport with this patient simply by treating him as a responsible citizen instead of as the fool of the family, and he responded well to psycho-therapy although he had no insight into the mechanism of his attacks. He was ready to accept a change of environment which subjected him to less strain, and on leaving the army became an assistant on a dairy farm where it was hoped he would be able to succeed in handling a job within his mental capacity.

The technique of treatment is one of moulding circumstances to suit the patient as he himself is unchangeable. Some are of course quite incurable and it is a waste of one's time to try and help them. The monthly sick paper delivered as quickly as possible is the best way out.

B.U., a man of 40, was a frequent attender at the surgery. He was unmarried and when his mother died he developed pains in his stomach and became an expert at aerophagy. He broke the monotony of belching by having a hysterical collapse, and occasionally lost the power of speech. He was investigated at the local hospital with negative results, but he remained worried and complaining. He was referred to the R.M.O., but he had a convenient "fit" en route and was taken to hospital instead. Rehabilitation was suggested, but his symptoms at once became worse. The only way out is to see him as little as possible when he comes for his sickness certificate. These are the kind of people who do live perpetually on one's doorstep ; but it is a mistake to think this applies to all functional cases. They only form a small proportion of the whole.

Gross hysteria can be a prelude to a psychosis. This was illustrated in the case of J.B. described in the last chapter, where a hysterical collapse was the first sign of a presenile psychosis.

Mrs. P.A., a woman of 47, came to see me in a great state. Her mother-in-law was interfering in her house. She poured out a long story of grievance. Her husband was epileptic and she had been deceived about this when she married. He was unable to work and she wanted to get a job but her mother-in-law would not co-operate by helping her out. It was a long and tearful story. The next day was her wedding anniversary. She went for a walk with her husband, and at two o'clock, twenty three years from the time of her marriage, she began to behave in a strange way. Her husband had difficulty in getting her home. When I saw her the day following she was in bed. She was noisy, emotional and resistive. She would answer no questions, but amid storms of tears she told me her children had turned against her. Then she would smile happily and say all would come right, as God had revealed it to her. She would co-operate in nothing and refused her food. I certified her and sent her to a mental hospital. The dramatic sudden onset at the exact time of her marriage made me feel she was hysterical, but it was in fact a prelude to a severe chronic paranoid schizophrenia. She has been in hospital now for four years and there is little hope of ever getting out again.

J.M., a man of 24, was another difficult case which at first seemed hysterical, but turned out to be an organic psychosis. He was a soldier with an I.Q. of 75 and had served a term of active service. After home leave he was put on a refresher course with a view to further active service, and at once began to throw fits. He said he felt queer and sometimes fell down but never actually lost consciousness. He never hurt himself, bit his tongue or passed water on these occasions. There seemed a motive behind his attacks and they were unlike true epilepsy. He was referred to us as a hysteric and on routine examination his W.R. was positive and his C.S.F. was typical of a G.P.I. Soon after admission to hospital he developed a cerebral thrombosis and hemiplegia. This slowly recovered but he became a typical dementia paralytica. He was slovenly in his habits, and his memory was seriously impaired. He was silly and facile and would burst out laughing for no reason. He was transferred to a mental hospital for malarial treatment.

The way in which hysterics can mislead one is illustrated in the following case:—

On reaching the surgery one night I found a small crowd round the back of a lorry in which lay a girl of 9. She had been found lying by the roadside. She could not be roused but resisted when one tried to open her eyes. My first impression was that she was not really unconscious, but was putting it on. I could not recognise her, but one of the spectators told me who she was, and then I realised she was epileptic. She was sent home labelled as a post epileptic state. I saw her mother the next day, and asked after the child. "I was waiting for her", she said, "she had taken some money out of my bag"!

Gross hysteria can usually be recognised with ease, but the hystero-anxiety takes more time. The whole group are troublesome and tiresome patients and while one cannot change their attitude to life one can persuade and cajole most of them back to work and a reasonable state of health, but medically they are unsatisfying and unprofitable patients.

REFERENCES

(i) Ross, T. A.   The Common Neuroses.   1937.
(ii) KRAINES, S. H.   The Therapy of Neuroses and Psychoses.   1943.
(iii) BARBOUR, R. F.   Modern Practice in Psychological Medicine.   1949.

CHAPTER X

RARER FORMS OF PSYCHIATRIC ILLNESS

Schizophrenia

SCHIZOPHRENIA is the most tragic of all mental illnesses. A depressive breakdown is distressing but a schizophrenic breakdown is even worse. It occurs in a younger age group and the prognosis is much more unfavourable. Henderson and Gillespie (i) write as follows :—

"It is now generally recognised that although the schizophrenic type of disturbance *is always serious**, there are certain cases which can and do readjust themselves. There are a large number who make a social rather than a complete recovery. **The vast majority do gradually show a state of mental deterioration, which particularly involves the emotional fields, and such patients are best cared for under mental hospital conditions.*"

The disease is of unknown ætiology. It usually attacks the solitary, withdrawn and eccentric personality, and no particular social stratum is immune. Intelligence is no deterrent to the disease. Not infrequently a young person who is quite brilliant at school falls a victim, and the family who imagined they had a genius in their midst have to watch with heart-rending sorrow their hopes fade as mental deterioration sets in. One parent told me pathetically, "We will have to reorient our whole lives now, to do what we can for what can be saved from the wreck".

The patient is usually a shy retiring person, who prefers his own company and avoids the crowds. One is nearly always called in to see the patient by anxious relations, who have noticed a change, but they sometimes shut their eyes to the early symptoms hoping they will pass off. Such is the fear of

*Italics ours.

mental illness and its dreaded implication, the mental hospital, that relations may hold back from calling in the doctor. Any strange behaviour is put down as mere eccentricity, or sheer bad temper. The schizophrenic rarely seeks advice on his own account. He tends to enjoy the world of make-believe he is building round himself and he resents interference from the outside. In this he is very different from the depressive, who knows he is ill, and usually seeks help in spite of feeling hopeless. The grosser psychiatric symptoms such as ideas of reference, delusions and hallucinations are more common among schizophrenics, than in other mental diseases.

This type of illness creates an atmosphere of its own. Relations often point out significant changes which the doctor cannot see for himself unless he knows the patient very intimately. The patient himself often feels changed and will admit he is a different person from what he was. Occasionally he describes himself as two persons. "Sometimes I am myself, but more often I am some strange new creature", was how a patient depicted his feelings. Like the depressive he shows no real interest in the psychiatric approach, and he feels emotionally empty. If he cries, his tears are crocodile in character. They lack the emotional quality of true depression or sorrow. A show of tears may give way to a fatuous smile, but the grossly depressed schizophrenic may be difficult to differentiate from a true melancholic. Such patients **are** often intensely suicidal. The tremendous power and the urge was illustrated in a patient who hanged himself in a lavatory. He had to hold his feet off the ground voluntarily as he could find no gallows high enough for the usual jump, from which there is no return.

Modern treatment in the form of insulin therapy, electronarcosis and leucotomy have much improved the outlook, but all authorities are agreed that early diagnosis and early treatment give the most hopeful results. This throws a great responsibility on the general practitioner. He must be able to pick out the schizophrenic from other psychiatric conditions, and refer him to a psychiatrist as soon as possible. Schizophrenia has been aptly described as the surgical emergency of psychiatry. The sudden violent catatonic types are easy to diagnose, but the insidious hebephrenic or simple schizophrenia can easily be missed. It is not in the province of this book to give a detailed description of schizophrenia, but rather a few salient points which help to make the early diagnosis, and the first point is to be aware of the importance of catching it early, and to be constantly on the lookout for schizophrenia among the army of functional cases. If in doubt the opinion of a psychiatrist should be sought at the earliest opportunity.

E.B. was a youth of nineteen. I was called in to see him by his mother. I found him sitting by the fire with his head in his hands. He complained of a headache, but on examination, I found no evidence of physical disease. His parents told me he had always been a quiet boy who only had one friend. Lately he had become very subdued, and even his solitary companion had no appeal. He just wanted to sit by the fire after his work and at the week-ends. The youth had a queer look in his eyes. When I asked him to tell me more about his headache, he said it was not really a pain, but a dead feeling, as if he had no brain. He had no interest in anything and he could not take his mind off his head. He felt he was changed in some way. He was full of queer feelings which were indescribable and very fearful.

He was quite willing to see a psychiatrist and the diagnosis of schizophrenia was confirmed. He was admitted to a mental hospital forthwith and after three months he was discharged as having recovered. He had had insulin and he assured me he was back to normal in every way.

For four years I followed him up and he remained well and at work, and then quite suddenly all his old feelings and fears returned. As is usual with a schizophrenic, I was sent for, and I persuaded him to go back to the mental hospital. Unfortunately on this occasion every kind of treatment failed to move his delusions, and at the time of writing leucotomy is under consideration. This quiet hebephrenic reaction carries with it a bad prognosis.

W.J. was a medical student of 19. I was asked to see him by a colleague as the youth had suddenly turned up at his home having cycled 130 miles or more overnight in appalling weather to see a football match. His host was a great friend of the boy's father.

When I saw the lad he was completely rational and quite prepared to talk. He was untidy and wore the sand shoes in which he had travelled. He stated that he just wanted to see a football match in this area, and he was fed up with his father who had been hard on him in money matters. He frankly admitted he could spend £100 in a day, and that he had no head for finance. He had been to a public school and was far ahead of his age group as regards work. He passed his school certificate at 14 and had been top of his form. On the other hand he had recently failed his first M.B. examination. At 15 he failed in some athletic ambition and his nerves gave way. He had to be taken away from school, and was sent to a psychologist who looked after awkward children. He hated the man, quarrelled violently with his fellows and ran away. His parents had kept him at home and taken him for long holidays to rest his nerves, and a year previous to my interview he had started in a medical school. The work, he said, was easy. He was full of confidence, but could not explain why he had failed his examination. He was obviously an impulsive youth, and it was difficult to keep him to any point on discussion. There was almost a manic flight of ideas.

In a single interview I could make no diagnosis. I suspected either schizophrenia or psychopathy, both of which were beyond my scope. The sudden change of character at 15 suggested the former diagnosis.

I told his friends that he should see a psychiatrist as soon as possible. The following week-end the boy's parents came to see me. I told them the boy was ill and needed urgent psychiatric attention. I was asked if I thought he was insane ; and I replied that it was obvious to all that his behaviour was irrational at times. The parents obviously resented the suggestion of a mental illness and were loathe to risk seeing a consultant in case "it would put ideas into his head". Reluctantly they agreed to my suggestion but vowed they would never let him "go away". I suggested that a psychiatrist might want to observe him and test him out in various ways, and that hospitalisation in some form would be necessary.

He saw a specialist who advised that he be admitted to a private mental hospital for observation. This advice was at first declined. He was taken to Ireland for yet another holiday where he started a violent love affair with a most undesirable girl. His parents consulted some medical relations who strongly supported the course which had already been suggested. Reluctantly they agreed and after a month of observation the verdict of hebephrenic schizophrenia was given, with a poor prognosis.

This case illustrates how the taboo of mental illness can affect parents. In their hearts they were worried, but rather than face facts, four precious years were wasted before even a diagnosis could be made.

The following case is an example of the acute explosive type of schizophrenia which is rarer, but is more easy to diagnose.

J.M., a boy of 22, complained of pains in the head. I could find no signs of physical illness, indeed he had been working until the day on which I saw him. His parents stated that he had not been himself for a week. He was a quiet boy as a rule, but recently had become aggressive and bad tempered. He had ideas of reference, in that he felt the men at work were talking about him. He admitted his headache was not real pain, but rather an inability to think. I gave him a sedative and promised to call the next day. I was sent for the same evening. He was very confused, was talking to himself and became violently aggressive when crossed. He was certified and sent to a mental hospital where he had a course of insulin treatment. He was discharged three years ago and has been well and at work ever since.

Admission to Mental Hospitals

Hospital treatment is essential for all schizophrenics and it seems convenient to discuss here the problem of sending patients into a mental hospital.

They can enter an institution either voluntarily, when they can leave at 72 hours notice : or they have to be certified. If the latter course is taken they lose their liberty and they have no powers to refuse any treatment thought necessary by the hospital authorities. The general practitioner has to decide under which category the patient will be admitted. Voluntary admission is desirable whenever possible, but the patient must be the right type and he must be prepared for the ordeal. It is a waste of everyone's time and most upsetting to the hospital staff if a voluntary patient gives in his notice after a few days. He usually airs his views about the institution, views which are far from complimentary ; he boasts that he still has his liberty and can leave when he wishes, and so greatly upsets those fellow sufferers who stay behind. The disease of "handing in one's notice" is infectious, and if one voluntary patient walks out, others usually follow him. Thus it behoves the general practitioner to consider very carefully whether or not the patient has the necessary personality to see the ordeal through. If he raises a series of objections to going away, and is not likely to settle, then he should be certified. The main groups of patients requiring such a course are schizophrenics and hysterics. A depression in a good personality type who knows he is ill can usually be sent as a voluntary patient. If however he is also a hysteric, he will not settle and should be certified.

The general practitioner's proper handling of the case prior to hospitalisation will go far to make the sojourn there more pleasant and helpful to both the patient and the staff. *No patient however foolish, difficult or demented should ever be tricked into going to a mental hospital.* Whether as a voluntary patient or under certificate, both the sick person and the relatives must be told he is going to a mental hospital and the hospital must be named. If he doesn't like it he can protest, but he cannot claim to have been cheated or deceived. It is a fearful experience for a patient to be told he is going for a ride in a car, only to find himself driven into a mental hospital to be locked up. He then has every right to be indignant and unco-operative. His faith in the medical profession is broken and a good rapport, the basis of all sound psychiatry, may be very difficult to resurrect. If he goes to hospital protesting violently but knowing the truth, rapport can be established quite readily at the other end. He has been made to take a dose of very unpleasant medicine by his doctor; but he has not been deceived. When he returns from the hospital he rarely bears any resentment.

Persuasion is part of the psychiatric art, and in my experience, although one often anticipates difficulty and even violence in getting a patient off to hospital, it very rarely happens. Once one has made up one's mind on the correct course of action, the family must first be consulted. I make it a rule that a patient is never sent away without the full consent and approval of the near relatives. They are usually easy to win over. It might be necessary to certify a patient who was dangerous to himself or others, against the wishes of his relations, but so far I have never had to do it. If the subject is approached tactfully, the family usually become most useful allies. In most cases it can be explained that the patient is going to hospital for treatment with every hope of recovery. The family usually know of other cases in the practice who have gone away and come back cured. These examples are a great help both to the practitioner and to the family. Having won the family over, all preparations are made for the patient's transfer to hospital and then before he actually goes, he is told why he is being sent away and where he is going. It rarely happens that one has to get a patient to hospital at the first interview. Even if hospitalisation is urgently needed it is usually possible to get in one or even two interviews, in order to make a diagnosis and establish a good rapport.* Once the latter has been established, one can order the patient to obey with considerable authority as a good father. With those who can reason, I use persuasion; with those who cannot reason I give orders and refuse to argue. I tell them I know what is best and that what is being done is for their own good. I often see my patients into the ambulance myself, if necessary persuading and encouraging them all the time and so far I have had no violence and no great difficulty.

Paraphrenia

This condition is one of the systematised delusions with hallucinations. It is a rare condition in general practice.

Mrs. A.W., aged 39, had been a mental nurse before the war. Two years prior to my seeing her she had lost her husband in the Air Force. She was a telephone operator in the army. One night in her own house, the dog started barking and she saw three men peering at her through the window. When she asked them what they wanted, they just laughed. She was not afraid, and just went off to bed feeling annoyed about it. These men and many others annoyed her by peering through the window, or by following her in a motor-car. They would hoot at her and then drive off laughing. She never managed to hear what they said except on one occasion when a voice shouted at her "Don't drink that"! She decided to pay no attention as it was just another of her persecutors' tricks. She could describe these men clearly ; but the police could never find any evidence that her persecutors were real. She had no insight into her condition, and life became so difficult for her that she was sent to a mental hospital.

A woman asked me to see her husband W.B., a man of 48. She was very worried about him as he was sure he had a cancer in his mouth and he refused to see a doctor as he was convinced his condition was hopeless. He was rather annoyed

*However psychotic the patient seems at the first session, if possible see him again before certification. I have seen a typical picture of schizophrenia clear overnight, and found myself faced with an apparently normal person the next day.

when I called in to see him. I told him that his wife was very worried about his condition and that was why I had called—in an effort to help her as well as him. He told me he had a growth and I was too late to help. He let me look at his mouth which was badly ulcerated as he was burning up "the cancer" with acetic acid. This he assured me was his only method of keeping the tumour at bay : "but it would get him in the end". In my visit I humoured him in every possible way in order to make rapport and before I left he agreed to visit me at the surgery. He never asked me what I thought about his method of treatment and I suggested nothing as I felt argument might antagonise him. He had made it quite clear that acetic acid was his only hope.

At the surgery he told me that his "cancer" was a judgment on him, as he had once bet on dog races—and betting was against his principles. He slept well and did not appear depressed. He was at work doing quite a responsible job in a coal mine.

In the end I told him I could quite see his point of view ; but I did not agree with it. As our opinions differed I suggested a third party in the form of a specialist should be seen ; and so I manœuvred him into seeing a psychiatrist. The latter in addition to my findings elucidated all kinds of auditory hallucinations ; but they were not very clear, and I would have described them as mis-interpretation of sounds rather than true hallucinations. The psychiatrist gave a very bad prognosis, and advised me to keep him at work as long as possible. More courageous than myself, he advised the patient to leave off the acetic acid, as it was injuring his mouth. To my surprise he gave it up and in a few weeks his mouth ulcers healed. His delusion of cancer cleared, and he remained fit and well for 2 years, only to fall victim once more to his systematised delusions, and he reverted to the acetic acid treatment.

Paranoia

This rare and apparently hopeless psychosis consists of carefully systematised delusions of persecution without hallucinations. It is a "mono-mania" and at once the patient is the least mad and the most mad of all psychotics. In relation to his delusions he is hopelessly insane, but in every other way he is completely normal.

A man W.J., aged 40, came to see me with a black eye. He stated his wife was carrying on with a taxi driver. He had missed her one night and went to look for her. A taxi passed him on the road. After a fruitless search he went home and found she was back before him. She had not passed him on the road, and could only have gone home in the taxi. He admitted he had no real proof of her infidelity ; but he was quite convinced of it. His wife still continued to have sexual intercourse with him. She had not denied him that.

When I asked him why he had approached me on the matter, he said his wife had sent him. I spent 20 minutes talking to him that night and I decided he was a possible paranoia. What guilty wife would ask a third party to intervene ? I asked him to send her along and a pitiful story she had to tell.

For the past two years he had grown more and more suspicious of her, until every movement and every act had some subtle significance. If she glanced at the clock, she was working out the time of a rendezvous ; if she rustled some paper, it was a note. If a car hooted in the street it was a secret sign. He followed her everywhere, spying on her, hiding behind hedges, etc., in order to obtain positive proof of what to me was clearly a delusion. On one occasion her husband had threatened her with a knife, and I felt he might do her grievous harm. I asked her to stay with her family until I had seen him again.

He was a bit upset by his wife's absence but I told him I had advised her to stay away until we had settled the misunderstanding. To my surprise he admitted he might have misjudged her ; and he promised if she came home, he would never speak about the matter again.

I saw his wife the next day and she agreed to go home: but of course after a few days, back came all his delusions and his unpleasant insinuations. He became worse than ever so his wife told me, and I arranged to see him with a psychiatrist.

Like most of the "Schizophrenic group", at first he resented the intrusion, but he was easily persuaded to speak his mind in the whole matter. He told us how her paramour used to park his car on a main road a mile away and flash signals with his headlights. It is curious how completely rational in some ways these psychotics can be. He noticed someone had inscribed PET in the flyleaf of a library book. A few days later he saw some birthday greetings in the personal column of a local paper signed PET. As it was not his wife's birthday, he was sure it was her paramour's, so he made it his business to run into this man's sister. "How old is your Bill?" he asked, "I am sure he is younger than I am". "He is 35 on 5th November" replied the woman. "I knew I was right", he said. He had the information he required, but as it was then March, it was obvious the birthday greeting wasn't what he had thought it was. He had the reason and logic to agree that his search had ended in a blank. The psychiatrist endorsed my views and suggested certification. Viewing the case from the general practitioner's point of view it is extremely difficult to know what is the right course to take. The man has never lost a day's work and apart from his system of delusions is perfectly rational. Certification means inflicting a life sentence on him as there is no treatment which will cure paranoia. Why should he be so condemned and why should the community be burdened with yet another expensive inmate of a mental institution, when he is perfectly capable of earning his own keep? The obvious solution appears to be a legal separation which would put the wife beyond his reach, but apparently this can only be achieved, if medical evidence is withheld (in which case the father keeps the only child), since apparently a husband who is insane and perhaps dangerous may not legally be deserted ! The handling of such a case with fairness and humanity is one of the most difficult problems in psychiatry.

Obsessional Neurosis

This condition is one of the most trying of all the neuroses. Fortunately although it resists psychotherapy, it is often relieved by the surgeon's knife, as it is in this type of case that prefrontal leucotomy does most good, especially if the obsession is accompanied with anxiety. In four years I have had two such cases. Mrs. E.F., aged 42, came to see me because her stomach was too big. The girls at work made fun of her and told her she was pregnant. Examination revealed a mutilated body. She had had her left breast off for some simple tumour and "everything removed"* because of a uterine fibroid. Both lumps had clearly been simple tumours but she had been convinced they were cancerous and she had willingly undergone operations for their removal. For 15 years she had lived in fear of cancer and she openly admitted she was sure her abdomen was swollen because she had a growth. Her anxiety was pathetic and she often told me with tears how bad she felt about it all. Every spot, pain or sore was a new cancer in her mind. Her I.Q. was probably very low and psychotherapy was not attempted. She was referred to a psychiatrist to ask for leucotomy. He agreed to the idea, but felt she was a poor personality type and not a good subject for the operation. However at my request she was referred to a neuro-surgeon. He too was diffident, but fortunately the patient was willing for anything and she had a unilateral leucotomy performed. That was three years ago. She took six weeks to get back to work after the operation, and has remained at work ever since except for an occasional week or two on the club; the amount of illness one would expect in a high grade mental defective. The only major symptom is a persistent and intractable polyuria, which gets her out of bed 3 or 4 times at night. She is still an anxious individual, but much easier to handle than before. I have never heard her speak of her stomach or a cancer. She is more cheerful and I have never seen her in tears since the operation.

*Patient's statement.

Her husband, who is a complete moron, and in a chronic depressive state following a head injury, is not very pleased with the result, if he ever gives his mind to think about it. She answers him back now, and when he asks her to do things she tells him sharply to do it himself, whereas before she was the complete doormat.

Friends from the factory say she is much happier, does not brood and never talks of her troubles. She was very touchy about her appearance before the operation, but one day soon after she had returned to work looking like an ex-convict with her close crop, she brought me a note which had been passed to her. It suggested she needed a "bubble-cut" and she fully appreciated the joke. Taking all in all I think the operation has been a success. Her anxiety is not fully allayed as she often comes to the surgery, and her polyuria is a real trial to her, but she is happier, and less anxious and can work instead of being a burden to the community.

In this case both the psychiatrist and the neuro-surgeon were reluctant to operate on such a poor personality type. The operation is at present largely confined to difficult and hopeless psychotics in the mental hospitals, and to good personality types, which in psychiatry always give the best results no matter what the treatment. I feel there are probably many chronic sufferers who are condemned to lives of abject misery, who might benefit from the operation, but they never get past the general practitioner's consulting room. They are labelled as troublesome neurotics and left to manage as best they can on placebos. With a better understanding of psychiatry at general practice level, and with more active co-operation between the consultants and the general practitioners, many such patients could be largely relieved of their sufferings.

Psychotherapy for the obsessional must be deep to be effective and general practitioners are advised to pass such cases on to the expert. Sometimes one cannot escape seeing these people and attempting some psychotherapy in the hope of persuading them to accept more radical treatment. The following case is however an example of the futility of psycho-therapy in such people. In all I have given her 25 psychiatric sessions, and today she is as bad as ever she was.

Mrs. M.G., aged 34, was first seen in May 1947. She was a married woman with no family. She felt she was not fit to have a child of her own. She complained of lack of energy, brooding on what people said to her, slowness at work and inability to concentrate. She had felt much the same on and off since she was 16. At this age a boy had kissed her, and made improper suggestions to her and she had become obsessed for some months, with the idea that she was pregnant. She slept fairly well and had a normal appetite. The diagnosis appeared to be between anxiety state or endogenous depression and she was referred to a consultant. His diagnosis was a severe chronic anxiety state in an obsessional type. He ended his letter to me saying, "She will be a very tough problem to cure. Were this condition to continue for many more years one might have to think of a prefrontal leucotomy". How right he was.

Simple psychotherapy met with some initial success and I did not see her from October 1947 until January 1949, when she came along in a panic because she thought she had a goitre. I reassured her and in March 1949 the trouble really started. She had missed a period. I had an Asheim Zondek performed. It was negative. At three months I examined her, and she was obviously not pregnant. Then she had a period. None of these things helped her ; she had to see a gynæcologist—but even he could not reassure her. For nine months she remained convinced she was pregnant. I gave her several psychotherapeutic sessions with free association but it was useless. When no baby arrived in October she had a short respite and then she came back with trouble in the vulva. She was sure her husband had injured her with sexual intercourse. There were a few tags of torn hymen : but she would not be satisfied. Hymenectomy was performed ; but it was quite useless. In December 1949 she was still very troubled but she had ceased worrying me. In May 1950 I was sent for, and she had an acute appendicitis. I was amazed at her condition. She was an educated woman with fine working class parents ; but her home was filthy. She herself could never have washed or bathed for months. The bedroom was a shambles. I thought to myself as I looked at her she was nearing the border line of a psychosis.* Her husband burst into tears when he told me how helpless she had become. She would do nothing but sit about and talk of her "imaginary" troubles. She went to hospital for an appendicectomy and she returned still quite convinced there was something wrong although every doctor and nurse had been asked to have a look—and each had attempted reassurance.

The psychiatrist's suggestion of physical treatment seems the obvious solution ; but the family are bitterly opposed to it in spite of the degradation of her present way of life, the discomfort and misery caused to her husband and the mounting score of wasted hours spent by me in futile psychotherapy.

In spite of the bad prognosis occasionally one gets an obsessional who responds rapidly and unexpectedly.

B.A. came to see me complaining of a modest cold in his head. He was agitated and obviously very worried about himself. He fiddled with his fingers, mopped his forehead and blew his nose repeatedly. His record card showed that he had never seen a doctor for 15 years. Rather apologetically he asked if he could be put "on the club" for a few days, an unusual request with a common cold. He had no temperature, and physically he looked well, but he was clearly very tensed up. When pressed for further symptoms he said he had been run down for some weeks and was unable to sleep. He had queer suffocating feelings in his throat, especially at night. When I suggested that his nerves were all on edge he readily agreed. I pointed out how worry was usually the

*She has been seen by a second psychiatrist who disputes the diagnosis of obsessional neurosis. He thinks she is a chronic endogenous depression: but she still refused all forms of active treatment.

cause of "nerves" or anxiety, and after a little time he told me it wasn't really the cold that worried him, so much as the fact that he had lost his sense of smell. With encouragement he told me that for years he had suffered greatly, because at times he was aware that he emitted an unpleasant odour from his groins. As long as his nose was functioning he could detect the smell, but now that he had a cold, he had lost his defense mechanism, and could not take adequate precautions. He admitted that he felt quite desperate about it at times and had discussed his worries with no one but his wife. With his permission I saw her, and a strange tale she had to tell. She could never detect any smell, but at times her husband nearly sent her crazy. He was forever having his clothes washed and his suits cleaned. During the war when there was clothes rationing, life was well-nigh impossible, because he would not wear his old suits and new ones were of course, unobtainable.

When I saw the patient again he was very relieved to have found someone to whom he could talk. It did not take long to discover the source of his smell. It was the odour of semen which was so upsetting to him, and his fears went back to childhood practices of masturbation. He was also a latent homo-sexual, who, although married, rarely indulged in sexual intercourse, and when it did happen he felt polluted for days afterwards. He had no family, and wanted none to grow up like him.

Typically obsessional in make-up, he was hardworking and fastidious. He had lived with his fears and feelings of guilt for twenty years, without letting them get him down, but he was near to breaking point when I saw him. Both the patient and his wife were quite sure he was going insane. Some five sessions of psychotherapy gave him considerable relief. They in no way changed his obsessional make-up or his homo-sexual bias, but they relieved tension, made him feel better and made him easier to live with. His wife was quite delighted with his progress and the improvement.

Mania

This is much less common than the depressive version of the manic-depressive psychosis. A number of depressives pass through a stage of reactive euphoria following a depression. This is only the natural result one would expect from any patient who finds himself free at last from unpleasant symptoms. A minority pass through a stage of true mania or hypomania. One depressive who had recovered was visiting the chemist. The article she had asked for was in the window, and he asked her to reach it over herself. She was clumsy and brought half the contents of the window down, breaking quite a number of items. She was a quiet sensitive woman who would have been horrified by such clumsiness under ordinary circumstances, but in her manic mood she saw the funny side of everything and, as she explained to the astonished chemist, she "just had to laugh".

Cases of acute mania are readily diagnosed and need to be certified as they are quite unsuitable for treatment outside an institution, but they are rare. I have only seen two cases in the past four years. Chronic cases may be quite well able to look after themselves and cause no trouble in the community even when very psychotic.

Mrs. E.H., aged 76, has had manic bouts for the past 40 years. She is in a stage of mania for about 6 weeks in every six months. In between times she is a quiet retiring old lady, and when she is manic she evidently knows she is ill because she visits me daily during this phase. She talks incessantly and never answers any questions I put to her. I have never succeeded in examining her, as if I suggest it she leaves the surgery at once. The suggestion is a good way of getting rid of her, but she rarely stays more than five minutes. She never waits her turn but comes straight to my consulting room, knocks at the door, and waits impatiently until I dismiss the patient I am seeing. It would be useless to argue with her as she never listens to anything I say. I tried to write down her spate of conversation one morning and it went as follows :—

"I have a cardigan on this morning and I am clothed for the Autumn. You don't want to hear local gossip. It was 75° this morning. It's the harvest festival on Sunday. Mrs. W. will be presiding. Only one of my tomatoes was bad out of five. My sister was a servant when she came here. Some fun about the Russian atom bomb. They love playing with radar. I was anæmic when I was young—good morning". There is nothing I can do to help her, except listen to her remarks. After a bad week or two her visits grow less frequent and I know she is improving; and then she ceases to come for a few months while the mania is in remission. Even in her worst phases she wastes less of my time than many patients who visit the surgery with colds in the head and other untreatable trivialities. The community easily tolerates her in her difficult phases and enjoys her when she is well, so there appears to be no indication for certification and institutional treatment in this and similar cases. In considering any form of hospital treatment in whatever type of case, physical or psychiatric, it does no harm to remember that it's an extremely expensive business and bankruptcy will be a poor return to the community for having some of its minor irritations removed or petty disabilities investigated.

REFERENCE

(i) D. K. HENDERSON and R. O. GILLESPIE. A Text Book of Psychiatry. 1943.

CHAPTER XI

THE WASTE PAPER BASKET

IN making a survey, a unit of service is defined as a consultation, a visit, or the repetition of some prescription. In the statistical section it was shown that 15 per cent of psycho neurotics seen in a year are incurable by any known method of treatment. These unfortunate people haunt the doctor's surgery year in and year out, seeking some relief for their multitudinous symptoms, and they waste a great deal of the doctor's time. They take up about 40 per cent of the units of service devoted to neuro-psychiatric cases. This means that these chronic patients make use of their practitioner three times more frequently than the acute and treatable cases, and it is not surprising therefore, that so many doctors avoid psychiatry like the plague. Worn down by a few chronic neurotics, the average doctor does not feel drawn to sympathise with any functional patient, in case he too becomes equally troublesome and persistent.

The previous chapters have been designed to show that this fear is unfounded. The acute case can usually be treated fairly easily and he then ceases to trouble his general practitioner. When he does come back to the surgery one can look him in the face and inquire about the old fears and phobias, without the dread of a further spate of neurotic symptoms. The illness can be discussed as one talks about a previous attack of pneumonia, or a broken leg. If the neurotic has not been radically treated, one tends to view each visit with apprehension, and the patient is discharged from the surgery with all possible speed. Even the most radical approach will not however prevent chronic cases from occurring and from forming a real millstone. They are an irritating burden to every general practitioner.

Inherited defects should be included among the chronic mentally sick, although they do not as a rule constitute a very troublesome group. Other chronic cases may be divided into those who find their neuroses too profitable ; those who, for a variety of reasons, have received inadequate treatment for their troubles ; and finally those who labour in such difficult conditions that recovery is virtually impossible.

Inherited Defects

This group includes the low grade intellects, epileptics and the psychopaths. It is frequently stated that the community contains no less than a tenth of mental defectives. In general practice the impression is that these figures are an exaggeration. However, many teachers who, in their pupils, see a fair cross section of the community agree whole-heartedly with the figure. The explanation for this divergence of views must be that in this age of full employment there is work for so many people that even the moron can find employment within his capacity, and so live a useful and healthy existence. In a large village of about 6,000 souls only a dozen cases of gross mental defect amounting to imbecility or idiocy were found. Two of the twelve were actually mongols who had augmented the numbers by an unusual span of life, since both were over 30 years of age, and they do not usually pass the second decade. This small group is a burden to their families and to the community as a whole, but not to the general practitioner. As a rule no one expects anything to be done for their mental health.

It was considered that a study of epilepsy was beyond the scope of this book. In the village mentioned above there were four people suffering from the disease and totally incapable of work, and also a dozen of working age who are fully employed and no burden to the community.

While the tenth of defectives is probably a fair assessment, the number of psychopaths is more difficult to estimate. They appeared more numerous in the army than in civil life, but that was probably because they often made use of the medical officers in their efforts to get out of the army or evade their duties in one way or another, and thus made themselves conspicuous.

A psychopath is described by Henderson and Gillespie (i) as a person who from childhood and early youth is habitually abnormal in his emotional reactions. He is an individual who has failed to develop socially and to mature emotionally. The intelligence may be normal or even above normal. Three types are described. The commonest form is the hysterical personality and this has already been dealt with. The second form is the psychopath with anti-social trends, the potential robbers, murderers and men of violence. They occur in all strata of society from leaders of nations, like Hitler, to the lowest thugs of the slums. This type of psychopath rarely finds his way to the doctor's surgery. He usually ends up in the police court. Most villages of the size mentioned have three or four people who are recognised as local scoundrels and who are regularly away serving terms of imprisonment. Very occasionally the general practitioner may be called upon to deal with such an anti-social psychopath by certification. As the patient is not insane but dangerous from emotional instability, the problem is no easy one to handle.

M.B., aged 30, had been blind from birth. Her I.Q. was average, she could read and write in braille, and for some years had worked at the local blind institution. She had a psychopathic personality and was given to bouts of temper when crossed, and she was liable to strike out violently on such occasions. The officers at the institution were models of patience and forbearance over her. They continued to employ her but placed her well away from the others so that she could be overpowered before she could do any damage to the other blind folk. These temper bouts were not common, but they were unpleasant and dangerous while they lasted.

Her mother, a widow, had remarried ; and M. hated and detested her step-father. She never ceased to chide and upbrade her mother for her remarriage, and life for all concerned was very difficult and unpleasant. M. then quarrelled violently with the foreman at the blind institution and refused to do any work offered to her and so she was given her notice. Resentful against everyone, she took it out of her mother and attacked her more than once. I heard the story of these attacks and saw the bruises. M. never denied them but said she had been provoked. I had various sessions with her and tried to see her point of view, but she continued to make life in the home intolerable and was so violent that I felt that murder might well be done. I approached a local J.P.* with a view to certification, but he was loath to act against a poor blind girl and without his authority my hands were tied. One night I was sent for in a hurry and I called for the J.P. on the way. When we reached the house, there was a crowd of neighbours outside, and they remarked to the J.P. "It's about time you came". M. had made a scene and attacked her mother. Fortunately no great damage had been done, and the J.P. agreed at last to certification. The solution is not a happy one but appears to be the only one available in the circumstances.

The third type of psychopath includes the sexually abnormal and this subject has already been discussed. It is difficult to assess accurately the incidence of these cases. Two profound male homosexuals, whose appearance and carriage is typical, exist in this practice. There are half a dozen others who are probably latent homosexuals. It is very rare for one to be approached medically on such problems.

Thus a few psychopaths of all kinds will be seen in general practice, but the only type who habitually worries his doctor is the hysteric and most of the chronic psychiatric cases are, in fact, psychopaths of the hysterical personality type.

The Profitable Neurosis

The Compensation Neurosis

Few people have the moral fibre to part with a symptom which is financially profitable to them. The typical compen-

*Justice of the Peace.

sation neurosis is common, and well known to every general practitioner. Two cases are perhaps worth quoting.

E.T.B., aged 38, came to see me complaining of a pain in his back. He said it was due to an injury he had a year before. This man was a miner, but did not look the part. He gave a double-barrelled name, unusual in this district, and he was decidedly overdressed for the country, immaculate in his black coat, striped trousers and a black Homburger hat. I found no abnormality on examination beyond hypertension, in spite of many protests on the part of the patient. His whole bearing reeked of psychopathy to me but I was new to the practice in those days and decided that before sending him back to work I would give him the benefit of an orthopædic opinion. I stated in my letter that I felt sure he was exaggerating and would like support in this view before signing him off his sick benefits. The diagnosis of a ruptured disc was made. He was given plaster jackets, and months at a rehabilitation course, together with all the physiotherapy available. After three years of loafing, during which he bought a car and was always better dressed than his physician, the orthopædic department decided that there was "a nervous element in his case" and that he was unsuitable for radical treatment. He was then awarded £1000 in damages for a very doubtful injury and he went back to work and was never seen again at the surgery.

T.P., a man of 50, fractured his pelvis in a mine accident. He was given lavish rehabilitation courses, but when he finally got back to work he could only do light work for 4 days a week. He had a splendid work record prior to the accident and had risen to the status of a shotfirer. Since the accident he had been of necessity "degraded to the ranks" and he was very depressed and miserable. I suggested he took a lump sum for compensation, but he dare not do it. A few months later he was forced to accept £1000 compensation and within a month he was back shotfiring. I have never seen him since except when he had shingles. This man's case was different from the first I described. He did have a serious injury, both physical and mental ; he was a superior type of working man, but even he could not resist the deadly lure of compensation neurosis.

Compensation neurosis is not infrequently misdiagnosed, being easily confused with a post traumatic psychosis.

A.W., aged 53, was injured on his head, side and leg in 1941. Up to that date he had a good work record but since then it was bad. He held odd jobs up to 1943 but has never worked since. He was depressed and miserable, full of complaints and at times suicidal. He could not sleep at nights without sedation. I had several sessions with him, but his trouble was clearly more psychotic than neurotic. Never once did he suggest or hint at compensation. I sent him to a psychiatrist who agreed with my diagnosis of post traumatic psychosis. A period in a mental hospital under E.C.T. and insulin had no effect. On my advice compensation was claimed and he was awarded £500 but this has in no way ameliorated his symptoms. At first this man looked like a compensation neurosis, and one doctor had labelled him as a malingerer. In actual fact he is in a chronic state of depression, traumatic in origin.

If ever a man is injured, his mind is damaged just as much as his body ; and it is every bit as important to treat the psyche as the soma. Orthopædic treatment without psychiatric assistance is often futile and a waste of everyone's time and money. All severe injuries and minor traumata which fail to yield to treatment should have a psychiatric assessment. If there is the loss of an eye or a limb, the compensation problem is fairly easy. If on the other hand the disability is largely psychological and compensation is right and proper, it should be paid once and for all in a lump sum. The accident has shaken the patient's confidence in himself and he must be forced to stand on his own feet, or to live on his hump. With such treatment the good personality type will make a good recovery. Weekly compensation for psychiatric damage is a most dangerous procedure. Many a decent fellow is rendered permanently neurotic by weekly compensation because his nerves were upset. The only hope of a real recovery is a prompt settlement on a "once and for all" basis.

Hypochondriasis (Primary)

Hypochondria is described as a fixed idea of ill health which no amount of reassurance or treatment will remove.

Clinically there are two types, one who enjoys being ill, and the other who is distressed and frightened by his symptoms. For want of a better name the former may be called primary hypochondriasis. It is a very rare condition and in my view it is a deep seated anxiety state which is too profitable to be relinquished. The secondary form is common. It is the termination of untreated or undertreated anxiety states and depressions. Hypochondria is sometimes the prelude to a severe psychosis. The venereal disease phobia case, which fails to respond to the treatment advocated in an earlier chapter, is a case in point. The fixed idea of his disease is hypochondria, and it is not infrequently the beginning of a severe endogenous depression.

The primary hypochondriac enjoys being ill. He takes quite a pride in his complaints and is willing to talk about them with obvious pleasure, to all who will listen to him. The love of bed is a useful guide to this condition. The neurotic or the melancholic does not enjoy being put to bed. The former feels it is a waste of time and the latter can brood more freely in bed than when he is doing something. The patient who revels in "a few days in bed" is usually such a hypochondriac.

Mrs. C.R. consulted me because she was short of breath and had various pains in her chest and neck. She was a woman of 60 and her symptoms came on at any time and were unassociated with exercise. A physical examination revealed no abnormality. When I tried a psychotherapeutic approach it was strongly resented. She requested to be sent to a famous London physician who gave her a complete overhaul with all accessories. He found nothing to indicate cardiac disease, but he felt suspicious of the neck pain. He recommended rest, diet and an imposing list of medicaments. The patient was quite delighted. "I *knew* there *was* something wrong", she told me. While I disagreed with the diagnosis, I must admit he did more good than I could myself. She wanted to be pampered and fussed and a four page letter from a London specialist was a very powerful weapon in her hands. Since then she has spent four happy years "wrapping herself up in cotton wool" and leading a semi-invalid existence without any obvious sign of cardiac embarrassment.

Chronic Psycho Neuroses due to Inadequate Treatment

Psychiatric conditions may not clear up for a variety of reasons. If the patient is a hysteric or has a low I.Q. treatment is likely to be difficult and recovery will be partial rather than complete. Elderly patients and those who have had their troubles for more than a year are not promising subjects for treatment. If the material is poor gratifying results are unlikely, but one cannot blame the art of psychiatry for being unable to make the proverbial silk purse from the sow's ear.

On the other hand plenty of good material is allowed to deteriorate because proper psychiatric treatment is not available when it would be most effective. Untreated depressions and neglected anxiety states are a fruitful source of pitiful secondary hypochondriasis.

Hypochondriasis following Endogenous Depression

H.P., a man of 40, came to see me with pains in his legs. He had a bilateral hernia and he was awaiting admission for operation. He was a poor personality type and had been more on the club than the average patient. There were no physical signs of organic disease beyond the hernia, and in a psychotherapeutic session he told me he had "strained himself" as a young man before he was married and had had a urethral discharge for which he was treated at the venereal disease clinic. He felt sure his symptoms were due to this "strain" and he had many subjective feelings in his genitalia and anus. Psychotherapy was of little avail, and he was sent to hospital where both physicians and surgeons agreed the case was functional. He was sent for soon after and had his hernia repaired. When he came home he was in a pitiable state. He could neither eat nor sleep, he was in tears all day, and on one occasion he begged me to put him out of it altogether. His wife was worried and distressed about him and I persuaded him to go to a mental hospital for treatment. E.C.T. improved him but after six sessions he felt better and handed in his notice. After a few weeks he went wrong again. With difficulty I persuaded him to go back for more treatment. He agreed after some delay, but the mental hospital refused to have him back, because he had been a troublesome patient. I was advised to certify him, but I could not find adequate grounds for such a course. This was over two years ago. He has never done any work since. He is full of symptoms for which there is no physical explanation, and his life is a burden to himself and to everyone else. His mother is an old woman of 75 who is just the same. She has seen a doctor every week for the past 25 years, and there is never any evidence of organic disease beyond a moderate degree of bronchitis. According to the patient she never had a doctor until "the change"; but she has had her full share of them ever since.

H.W., a miner of 50, had a fairly good work record until 1948. He had a severe cough and according to the patient he brought up enormous quantities of sputum every day. He had quite a severe degree of bronchitis and emphysema, but X-ray investigation revealed no other abnormality. I tried to explain the condition to him but I could not satisfy him. He was sure there was something else there. He could not rest at night for coughing and he was depressed and miserable. He was sure he was finished. He gave a history of a "nervous breakdown" in his twenties and he had been to a mental hospital. I decided the diagnosis was a depressive graft on top of a chronic bronchitis. He was seen by a psychiatrist who agreed, and he was admitted to a mental hospital for

E.C.T. As in the previous case he defaulted after a few treatments and has never worked since. He remains in a chronic depressed condition. It takes him half the morning to get his chest free, but by evening he is quite cheerful and can enjoy a game of dominoes at the local public house. He still feels there is some serious lung disease causing his trouble, and he has asked me if I could get one of them removed.

Hypochondrias following an Anxiety State

Mrs. J.E., aged 50, came to see me complaining of queer sensations in her stomach which made her feel unable to stand. She was fearful of being left alone, and although she lived only a hundred yards from the surgery, she had to be brought down and taken home again. She was obviously very anxious and apprehensive. A complete physical examination was negative and I decided to try psychotherapy.

She had been perfectly healthy until she was 35, when her husband had contracted an appendicitis and had to be rushed into hospital. The day after his return home she was shopping and while gazing into a grocer's window she had "a black out". She was helped home by some friends and the doctor was called in. She had never been the same woman since, and lived her life under the threat of another fainting attack, hence her fear of being left alone. I spent two sessions on her taking her history, but it was heavy going. She was clearly not very receptive. In the end she told me candidly that she did not think talking would help her and she preferred her bromide mixture. I must have made some rapport because she always comes to me for her prescriptions rather than my colleagues, but she relies not on my advice but on the medicine, as she assured me she feels awful if she has none in the house.

If this woman had been treated radically at 35, she might have mastered her feelings, but at 50 she is now a hopeless neurotic.

Cases such as this are common place in every practice. I have a dozen or more who are chronic attenders at the surgery. From an initial history one can see that they are too set in their ways to benefit by psychotherapy and I waste as little time on them as possible. For them a placebo is essential, but it should be kept as cheap as possible.

Chronic Neurosis due to Environment

The stress and strain of circumstances are the cause of all neuroses. One's first aim is to help the patient to face up to difficulties and if possible to master them. If this cannot be done, then one must attempt to "temper the wind to the shorn lamb". If this too is impossible then the case is incurable.

Miss B.F. was a woman of 40. Her illness started at 16 when spinal disease was diagnosed and she was put on her back for three months. Since that time she has always had a "weak back", although no G.P. or specialist has been able to explain the cause. From the psychological point of view she had enough to break anyone's back. She was an intelligent and very capable person, but at 14 all hopes of advancement along her own lines went when she was drawn into the family business because of her mother's illness. The family were thrifty and hard-working to a degree of absurdity. Work and money-making were the only things that mattered. Social life was frowned on ; smoking and alcohol were forbidden. At 40 her mother still referred to her as a young girl and treated her as such. After a few sessions there was a vast outpouring of hatred against her mother with floods of tears. After that she felt better but never completely well. How can she get well under such impossible circumstances?

For months I saw her periodically for a painful session of half an hour or more. She cannot improve because she is in a hopeless trap until her parents die, and she cannot stand on her own feet. By then it may be too late. She has not the training, resources or courage to go elsewhere. She cannot change either herself or her circumstances and so she remains a chronic and troublesome neurotic.

Chronic psychiatric cases of whatever group form a depressing array. They are to all intents and purposes incurable, and they constitute a serious social problem, as few of them are able to work regularly enough to support themselves and their dependents. Ways of averting the compensation neurosis have been suggested. With better psychiatric facilities and closer co-operation with psychiatric units, the incidence of chronic incurable psychoneurotics could be lowered.

A large proportion of this waste material is a result of endogenous depression. Earlier and more accurate diagnosis at general practitioner's level and better facilities for specialist treatment, together with a removal of some of the stigma that make it difficult for patients to accept treatment early, would materially reduce the number of chronic endogenous depressions. Similarly, if psychotherapy were more readily available, there would be fewer hypochondriacs from anxiety states to occupy our time and depress our spirits. There will however always be a residue of waste who can only be treated by placebo.

The Regional Medical Officer is sometimes a useful ally with these cases, as occasionally he can provide the general practitioner with the necessary lever for getting them back to work. Once in a while one is able to force the patient back to work by the blunt refusal of a certificate, and once coerced into employment he keeps away from the hard and unsympathetic surgery for considerable periods of time ; but alas, the bulk of these patients are always with us.

REFERENCE

(i) D. K. HENDERSON and R. D. GILLESPIE. A Text Book of Psychiatry. 1943.

CHAPTER XII

PROPHYLACTIC PSYCHIATRY

As the ætiology of the affective psychoses is unknown nothing can be done to prevent them. The best the family doctor can do is to look for the first symptoms of the condition and aim at early treatment. Prophylaxis in psychiatry is thus largely confined to the neuroses.

Anxiety states are brought about by the stresses and strains of environment. In adults the commonest cause of anxiety is frustration either at work or in the home. Difficulties in the work environment are often beyond the scope of the family doctor, but today many industries are sympathetic to the psychological approach. Where such is the case, with the patient's permission, the firm can be consulted and the problem alleviated. Care must be taken to sort out the genuine case who will benefit by such help, from the psychopath and hysteric, who is just out to exploit his symptoms for his own benefit. Insecurity takes second place in the causes of anxiety, and while the work situation may be the predominant factor as in compensation neurosis, most of the insecurity problems come from childhood and the home environment.

Realisation that the seeds of anxiety are sown in the early years of life underlines the importance of treating all cases of childhood neurosis, either at the surgery or by reference to suitable clinics. Many behaviour problems can be prevented by better education of the parents, and mothers in particular are eager to learn how to handle their children. Lectures on childhood problems are always in great demand by Women's Institutes and allied bodies. No opportunity to assist in this group prophylactic therapy should be lost. A small proportion of neuroses arise direct from sexual troubles, and feelings of guilt ; and these are essentially within the province of general practice. The vast majority of cases arise from the stresses and strains associated with the home and family life. Indeed a happy home life is the best antidote to most neuroses. The general practitioner is in a unique position to assist in the construction of such homes, if he accepts his responsibility to do so, and in this way he is going far in the direction of prophylactic psychiatry.

Pre-Marriage Guidance

Adults who marry in ignorance are often inhibited not only physically, but in their whole attitude to sex. They cannot teach their children what are commonly called the "facts of life" in a healthy atmosphere ; and a new generation of sexually ignorant and immature individuals arises. This vicious circle of ignorance and inhibition must be broken if the mental health of the community is to be improved. Parents with a strong taboo are poor instructors for their children. The teaching of sexual knowledge in schools has its own dangers and may be followed by a flood of juvenile experimentations. Instruction of adults themselves is often ineffective because they have often learned bad habits and are set in their ways. There is, however, one period in life when individuals are in a receptive mood when instruction, even if it stimulates desire, can do little harm, namely the period immediately before marriage. This is the ideal time for instruction not only on sexual matters, but on family life and the upbringing of children. Nowadays there are several excellent books on the subject, and few intelligent young people marry without some reading and mutual discussion. Mace (i) suggests this is not enough. He stipulates that book knowledge alone is insufficient and can never replace pre-marriage guidance. There are two good reasons for this. The instructor like the psychotherapist acts as a kind of catalyst. He may impart no new knowledge, but he assists in freeing the young people from inhibitions and accelerates the normal maturation of their attitude to sex. Secondly, those who are instructed feel they have a friend and mentor to whom they can refer should any unexpected difficulty arise.

In any form of sex instruction, the lecturer must be sufficiently free from inhibitions to put across his lesson without embarrassment. The family doctor whether he likes it or not is often faced with delicate situations. He may be confronted by the desperation of an unmarried mother or the frustration of a childless couple. He frequently has to ask questions and to talk about intimate subjects. The married doctor fortified by even an elementary knowledge of marriage guidance is an ideal instructor, and any inhibitions he may have disappear when his knowledge is turned by practice into experience. Living in a community in which he knows people intimately he has an opportunity rivalled only by the clergy in knowing who is preparing to be married and who to select for instruction. It is therefore urged that premarriage guidance is one of the most important functions of the general practitioner. This task may be fulfilled in a variety of ways. The method adopted here is described in some detail so that beginners may make use of it as they wish until, through experience, they have evolved a routine of their own, with no doubt many modifications and improvements.

Any young people who are about to be married are invited for an interview a month or two before their marriage. They can come separately or together as they wish. Unless they request it, no physical examination is advised. Practices vary, but this one is remarkably free from venereal disease ; only two positive Wasserman Reactions being known among 8,000 patients. Any useful information which might be gained by such an examination is more than offset by embarrassment, especially to the young woman. There is a feeling abroad that premarital instruction should consist of examination of the sex organs and instruction about the sexual act, and because of this many young people approach the matter with some distaste although, realising their ignorance, they feel it to be necessary. It is very important that they should be reassured and put at their ease before any intimate advice is given.

Good premarital guidance should encourage the couple to think about and plan their future and to make them realise that marriage is something worth discussing before they take the plunge. It makes a good opening to point out that young people on the verge of matrimony are about to embark on a new career, and that just as it takes five years to become an efficient plumber or any other artisan so it takes time and patience to make a satisfactory marriage. It is a fallacy to suppose that young people will fall into the art of married life by instinct. The couple should then be asked how many children they intend to have, whether they have made any plans or if they are going to be content with a series of accidents. It is worth while producing a theory of family planning and spacing at this point, not because there are any absolute standards in these matters but with a view to provoking thought and discussion. This plan should include a year of adjustment as a preliminary to a family of reasonable size and spacing.

The Year of Adjustment

However much people are in love with each other, adjustments have to be made once they are actually married. During courtship they look at things through rose-coloured spectacles. This is nature's way of drawing them together. Once they have been married for a few weeks, they lose their rosy spectacles and pass through a stage of reaction. If they have been told to anticipate this phase, it probably won't upset them. Most married couples pass through a period which is difficult until they get used to each other and the new way of life. If a baby is coming at this stage, it becomes a three cornered contest, and the shakedown period may be greatly prolonged. A pregnant woman is at a disadvantage. The young husband may be pressing his attentions on her and she may turn against his lovemaking and against him. So it is felt that the wise couple should plan a period of about a year in which no children should be conceived. It should be a kind of prolonged honeymoon, with plenty of sociability and entertainment, as this helps the settling-in process, Also once a family has arrived, the mother is tied to the home, and unless there is a good "sitter in" available, the couple will have few outings together.

If children are to be avoided, some form of birth control is essential. The couple should be advised that the practice of withdrawal, popularly known as "being careful", is a very undesirable and unsafe method of contraception. The sheath is probably the best method. It is easy to apply and very safe. In the early stages of marriage, as a rule, the man gets more pleasure out of sexual relations than the woman, and he should shoulder the inconvenience of taking precautions.

How Many Children

Most young people today realise that a single child is a mistake. They say the child is spoilt, which he often is, by too much undivided attention from his parents. It is also bad for the parents themselves as they are very literally "putting all their eggs in one basket". It is bad for the child because he is denied the privilege of other siblings who teach him the lessons which make him grow up a sociable individual.

The two child family is probably the popular favourite of today, but it is little better than the singleton for two reasons. Should anything happen to one child, the other is likely to be more spoilt and over protected than if he had never had a brother or a sister. Secondly, the unfortunate children have only each other with whom to quarrel. They often grow up intense rivals.

The three child family is the lowest reasonable family for a healthy couple; but it is the lowest and not the ideal. It is still too small, two children often tending to cling together leaving the third as an odd man out. So it is concluded that a four child family is the lowest ideal family. There are plenty of eggs in plenty of baskets and the children can pair off into a variety of ways for either aggression or friendship.

Spacing

The second child must not be born more than two years after the first. The closer the children are together the better for them unless the second child is more intelligent than the first when he may overtake his older brother at school and cause considerable embarrassment. The younger child has the advantage of an older sibling to copy which helps him to draw up to his rival. A two year start is usually sufficient, but parents should be careful not to treat the children as twins. The elder child must be given privileges for being the elder from the start, and these privileges must be maintained.

Opinion is divided on the spacing of subsequent children. There is something to be said for short spacing being maintained, so that all the family forms a single group but this makes for a period of intensely hard work for the mother. As an alternative it may be suggested that after a pair has been produced, they should reach the school age before the second pair is started, making life easier for the mother but thereby dividing the family into two groups. If only three children are contemplated, then the first suggestion is clearly the better.

In any case if a proper family is envisaged with reasonable spacing, the parents must be prepared to curtail their social life for a matter of some 15 years. This is not a long time, nor should it be in any way a sacrifice ; but it does underline the importance of a prolonged period of adjustment.

A common argument against the large family is the cost of education. Under the new education acts this argument is really no longer valid and in any case it implies a limited view of the subject. Crichton Miller has rightly pointed out that the most important part of a child's education is the first seven years in the nursery. That, of course, means having brothers and sisters to assist in the process of social adjustment.

Most couples enjoy a discussion on the size of a family and its spacing. They may quite well have started the session uneasily wondering, "What *is* he going to say". This introduction usually puts them at ease and once rapport has been established one returns to the importance of the year of adjustment. It is pointed out that contrary to popular belief, marriage relationship is not like putting a key in a lock, but it is more like playing a violin. Perfection is unlikely to come to them at once, just as they would be unlikely to master the art of the violin at the first lesson. They must be patient with each other and try to study each other's wishes and feelings. If all goes well, in six months to a year they will have mastered the art, which will never be forgotten and then they can start on the family. It is not necessary to go into more intimate details with a couple, or with a woman unless she asks for further advice, but it is advisable to give the man more detailed instructions such as can be found in any book on the subject. It must be explained that the male is more readily stimulated than the female and reaches his climax quickly, whereas his partner is likely to be slower and that the art of coitus is for both to achieve a climax at the same time. To begin with the young man must content himself with making love to his wife and exploring methods of stimulation. The erotic zones are mainly the lips, the breasts and the vulva itself. On the first night he should work up to the stage when he can explore the introitus digitally. Before the penis can be inserted, the woman should have started to moisten up in those parts, and he should be able to admit easily two or three fingers. During this early exploration he will probably have a climax, but that does not matter. The desire will return in half an hour or so and he can go a stage further. Intercourse should not be forced on the woman. The art of coitus for the man is to judge when she is willing to take him, to make love to her and to arouse her. Once fully aroused penetration is easy and he must learn to restrain his climax until he knows by the movements and excitement of his mate that she is reaching her orgasm. The penis should be kept inside until the woman's climax has passed off.

If a woman does require advice on these matters she is told that she needs more stimulation than her husband ; and that if he caresses her, this is a normal process. The sensitive vulva is there to be caressed. She is advised that coitus is an art, and if her husband is clumsy at first, she must be patient with him. She must however not rest content until she can obtain satisfaction. This is as much her right as her husband's. Two popular ideas need debunking. The first is that it is indecent for a woman to have feelings ; the second that if she does have feelings she will conceive. The second of these two ideas may make the woman hold back, because she thinks she is thereby preventing conception. The need for adequate birth control is thus underlined.

Marriage Guidance

This type of talk is designed as a pre-marriage instruction, but it can be used with a newly wed couple should such a pair seek advice. It is not altogether the content of the talk that counts. The couple are encouraged to think on these matters, and realise the importance of their new venture. Any plan of campaign is better than none at all and they are encouraged to work things out for themselves, but if things go wrong or they want further advice, they know where to find it.

In matters so closely linked with emotion young couples can be precipitated into very serious situations by their impatience and ignorance and saved by a little impartial advice and help, and they are themselves able to think more logically and less emotionally in the presence of a sympathetic but disinterested third party. This may be illustrated by the following case.

Mr. and Mrs. G. sought advice because they were not able to achieve proper coitus. They were in great distress and felt they were on the brink of a divorce. Each told his or her story separately and were then seen together. They knew the theory but failed in practice. They were told that their trouble was common place and that the only difference between them and other couples was that they realised the importance of such matters and had sought advice. It was suggested that they were in too much of a hurry and could not really hope to master the art of marriage in a few months. It was stressed that their trouble was not serious but was aggravated by their disappointment and anxiety. Nothing new was contributed to their knowledge but they were reassured that their troubles were in no way unique and would eventually be solved. Within a few weeks the husband reported that things were much better, and a year later they had their first child.

The next important occasion for prophylactic psychiatry with the young couple is when the first baby is expected. Busy general practitioners may find it extremely difficult to carry out the ritual of the Grantly Dick Read (ii) relaxation methods, but one can allay the great fear of the unknown if a little time is spent explaining to the patient what happens in labour, and how the doctor intends to help her. Read's use of the word contraction instead of pain is a great help. The idea that labour is a period of time during which the patient will be wracked with pains, mysterious, baffling and illogical, can only produce in her mind a state of fear. Some can control these feelings but they are always present. The idea of a strong purposeful muscular contraction which may incidentally be painful, can be accepted without panic because the process then appears to be reasonably planned and understandable.

The proper time to advise breast feeding is at the prenatal clinic. If one can induce the mother to accept the idea at that stage she will probably feed her own child. If one leaves persuasion until the puerperium when doubt has been inculcated by friends and relations, one is fighting a losing battle.

At the post-natal clinic every mother should be given explicit instruction on birth control, and before any method is finally chosen she is advised to discuss the subject with her husband. It should be explained that now she herself can be fitted with an appliance. She can be fitted by her own doctor at a special clinic or by a woman doctor if she so wishes. No chemical contraceptive on its own is really safe.

All contraceptive advice must be made very clear and every effort must be made to see that the patient really understands the instructions. It is amazing how crass the low grade intellects can be. One patient after her instruction asked if the cap had to be inserted before or after intercourse ! Another acquired a contraceptive sponge. The idea was explained and the sponge was inserted for her. Her adaptation of the method was to attach tapes to it and wear it like a sanitary towel, and nine months later she was rewarded with twins to augment a family of seven.

Sex Education of Children through their Parents

From now on an opportunity must be sought to see that the mother is educating her children properly as regards sex. In the standard family, the advent of a new baby should be the occasion for a lesson on the subject. All legends such as the stork and the doctor's black bag are strictly taboo. Children must be told the simple truth in words they can understand. These simple questions should be answered honestly and simply.

"Where do babies come from ?"

"They grow inside their mother."

"How do they get out ?"

"There is a special hole for them."

"Where is it ?"

"You know where you make water, there is a special opening for it. There is another opening you use when you go to the lavatory. There is a third opening from which the baby comes."

This simple story satisfies the child. His questions should be answered, but there is no need to go further than his questions.

Few intelligent young mothers today find difficulty in explaining parturition to their children, but the prospect of telling them about conception fills them with misgivings. The problem does not usually arise until the child is between 6–9 years of age. The growing child should be given opportunities of seeing these events in nature, and here the country cousin has a big pull over the town children.

They readily grasp the principles of pollination and the need for an admixture of both male and female seed. When dogs or cattle or insects are seen mating they should know what is happening. It should be as much a part of their mental furniture as the sight of a hawk hovering, or a dog chasing a hare.

Sooner or later comes the crucial question, "How do you and mummy mate ?" The child should be told that the principle is the same as in animals. The male seed is put inside the mother and the egg is fertilised. Precise details are unnecessary. If the child wishes to be a builder, the fact that houses are made of wood, bricks and mortar is of interest, but details of planning, foundations, how to mix mortar are unnecessary at his age. When he is learning his trade, he will have to learn these details. The same applies to sexual knowledge. It is right and proper to know the general principles, but the finer details can wait until he is of age to appreciate them. This should be explained to the child if he is pressing for further details and will be readily accepted : he should not be put off with untruths, nor made to feel he has asked a question which was improper.

Lessons in anatomy are as important as those on physiology. With a reasonable sized family where the sexes are mixed, all the members have ample opportunity at bath times for seeing things for themselves. At least until puberty is reached, there should be no locking of the bathroom door. The children should see not only their siblings but their parents. From time to time questions are asked, and usually they can readily be answered. "Why have you got hair there ?" "Because I am grown up. You will have hair when you are big."

Another useful point in the sex education of children is that they should learn the proper anatomical names from the start. It should come quite naturally for them to talk about the penis and the vulva. If they have learned these names in the age of innocence, they will use them without embarrassment when they are older.

No one likes children who are always causing parental embarrassment by talking sex in public. To safeguard this the childish love of a secret should be employed. The child is told that sex matters are a family secret. The family talk about such things together, but not with other people who are outside. If they do transgress this rule, strangers are usually very long suffering and tolerant on such matters, and the child can later be told of his error. He should not be corrected abruptly in public to make him feel foolish or guilty about it. Later he can be told quietly, "that's not the sort of thing we talk about with people outside the family". The secrets of success in sex education in children are honesty and patience. It should be started as soon as they are interested in such matters but there is no point in telling them the whole story at once. Answer their questions honestly, but avoid putting ideas for further questions into their minds. The younger the child the easier the task. The converse is also true. Puberty is much too late for sex education as far as parents are concerned and sex problems can then cause very profound anxiety states, and as the child is almost unapproachable their solution can be extremely difficult. I am indebted to one of my patients for the following history of one of his sons.

J.H. at 11 was a fat boy and apparently normal in every way. Suddenly he stopped eating and began to waste away. He saw specialist after specialist and, while all agreed his anorexia was functional, none could offer a solution or a cure, until the child's life was actually in danger. Ultimately a psychiatrist saw him and was able to probe into his mind and uncover a very simple problem.

The woman next door had been pregnant and was great with the child. J.H.'s friends had teased him and told him he too was pregnant. Terrified, he set to slim himself and very nearly killed himself in his efforts. It required very great skill to drag the guilty secret from him at that stage. Had he had the most elementary sexual knowledge the whole neurosis need never have happened. Boys and girls should be taught beforehand what changes to expect at puberty ; encouraged to welcome these changes as a sign of "growing up", and they should be prepared for any special problems associated with the period of change.

The chief problem of puberty as far as sex goes is that of masturbation, or as E. F. Griffith (iii) calls it, self stimulation. In the past this was considered to be verging on mortal sin and fraught with physical dangers. It was said to engender insanity and other fearful maladies if it continued unchecked. One patient remembers his mother telling him after she had caught him looking at himself, "There are worse things than stealing : there are worse things than murder". The truth is, of course, that masturbation is a natural phase through which all male children pass. Girls don't seem to be so universally afflicted with sex curiosity, and the desire to experiment and stimulate sexual feelings. The act of masturbation does no physical harm. Any damage lies in the realm of conscience. If the patient feels he is an addict to a sinful lust which he cannot abandon, and which is sapping his vitality, he is indeed in a bad way. Such feelings probably caused the suicide of a lad of 14 who was normal in everyway as far as was known.

C.F., a boy of 16, came to see me week after week with vague complaints. He had a sore throat, abdominal pain, headaches and there was never any clear organic basis for his symptoms. I saw him by appointment and explained to him the troubles of puberty. I did not ask him if he masturbated but I told him I knew all boys did. I explained that this had probably worried him and accounted for his vague complaints. I felt that the strain of puberty in a rapidly growing boy was making him body conscious and thus symptoms were provoked. He went home and told his mother the doctor had had an interesting talk with him and appeared to be much better, and ceased his visits to the surgery.

Boys and girls must be taught that such habits are likely to arise at puberty, and that the habits are bad ones only in the same way as it is ill-mannered to pick one's nose or bite one's nails, but no more serious ; and that if the habit is acquired it will pass over as one grows to the adult state. Good resolutions never cure bad habits. In fact as soon as the addict to any habit or craving swears he will never, ever indulge again, he is condemned to another fall and another chastisement from his injured conscience.

The general practitioner can help young folk through this awkward age in three ways.

(I) By seeing that the parents he has instructed do their duty by their own children.

(II) By undertaking to talk to children individually on such matters should the occasion arise, but at this stage it is important that the instructor should be the same sex as the child.

(III) By instructing classes such as at schools or churches should the opportunity for such instructions be given.

Self stimulation in adults is not uncommon if natural coitus is not available. It was used by soldiers abroad, and was much safer and more desirable than the brothel. "When I am at home my wife is my right hand. Now my right hand is my wife", was how one soldier explained it.

The community as a whole is profoundly ignorant of the problems of sex. G.P.'s can if they care to do so, go far to ease the communal burden in the matter, thereby engendering a higher standard of marital happiness and preventing unhappy marriages and psycho-sexual neuroses.

Neurotic parents produce neurotic children, not because of any inherited taint but because an environment of anxiety makes the child anxiety prone. This emphasises the importance of treating all neuroses in young people in a radical manner. The parent who has learned a little elementary psychology is probably better armed to face the battle of life than the parent who has never thought about such things.

Occasionally one has the chance of making a bigger contribution in preventative psychiatry.

A mother once told me she was worried about her daughter aged 21, as she was being courted by a very presentable young man, but would have nothing to do with him. The girl proclaimed she would never marry and looked forward to remaining a spinster all her life. I told the mother, I could only help her daughter if the latter agreed of her own free will to come and see me. Rather to my surprise she came along.

Miss L.P. was a very attractive young woman and she admitted she had a complete aversion to being kissed or touched in any way, and she had no interest in sex. I suggested that this attitude was unusual, and while at the moment it caused no great embarrassment, she might regret it later when it was too late to alter her way of life. She agreed to all this and welcomed my offer of psychotherapy.

She was the youngest of 4 siblings, having a sister and two brothers. She was only a moderate scholar at school, but had a good work record in 2 factories. She had chorea at 14 and was ill for six weeks. Her earliest memory was of falling into a brook for which she received a beating. Her bias was towards her mother, but she felt she was much too strict with the family. If quarrels occurred with neighbouring children, she was always beaten, and no effort was made to lay the blame fairly. Her older sister aged 32 was married with one child but was sexually frigid and unhappily married. In early childhood my patient had a crippled uncle living in the house. She was very fond of this man, and he was the only person in her life she could remember really loving. She enjoyed sitting on his knee and sharing his affection. She had another uncle who visited the house, and his approaches terrified her. As a child of five, she always felt he had an ulterior motive in his affection. She was always ashamed of her nakedness even as a small child. At eight a girl cousin was adopted. The other girl was 3 years older and the two became great confidants. They talked a lot about sex, but while my patient was interested, she never flirted like her cousin.

There was no evidence of early sexual trauma such as enemata or frights, except that as a child of 7 she fell on her perineum and bruised the vulva. A doctor was called in.

This girl had been starved of real affection. She had loved her crippled uncle but he died when she was seven. She was very tied to her mother for whom she had a great respect, but she had little love for her and never kissed her. Mother organised everything, buying her clothes and even choosing her boy friends. I encouraged her to be bold and "break" with her mother. This meant she had to grow more independent and she succeeded to some extent. On her own volition she decided to pay board instead of handing over her pay packet, and she started saving and buying her own things.

The whole business of sex was discussed openly with her. While she did not enjoy being kissed she admitted she was tempted to let men touch her breasts. This I pointed out was a natural urge, and showed she was not really as cold sexually as she imagined. In all, my therapy consisted of desensitising her to her mother and to sex as a whole. Three years have passed since I last saw her and in a follow up she wrote as follows :—

"I can honestly say you helped me a great deal. I am not married yet, but I hope to be soon". The final proof will only be forthcoming when she is married and has made a success of married life, but I feel I did help to steer her away from the previous negative attitude towards sex.

Family Problems

All marital difficulties are not tied up in sexual problems. The general practitioner is in an excellent position to give help when the stress and strain of double harness threatens the security of the family unit. In the statistical section it was pointed out that half the problems of frustration in marriage were easy to deal with, while half were serious. If the problem looks difficult, it is probably better for the couple to be referred to a marriage guidance centre, well away from the practice, so that their troubles can be aired in front of someone they will probably never meet again. Quite a number of cases can however be dealt with easily at the surgery.

Mrs. B.L. came to see me complaining of insomnia and being run down. She was in fact a mild anxiety state with depression. Once I had gained her confidence she told me the following story :— Her husband who was an overman at one of the local coalmines, was working for his undermanager's certificate. He was studying hard, and she was having to keep the family quiet all the time he was at home. They dare not even put on the wireless. I knew the family well, and I pointed out that her husband's ambitions were something to be proud of. The man had only had an elementary school education, but I learned from the schoolmaster that he had been a most promising scholar who really should have gone to a secondary school. After discussing the problem, I suggested to her that she should ask her husband to see me. I told her how I would talk to him, so that she would feel assured I would betray no confidence with her.

He came down a few nights later, and I told him that his wife was worried and depressed. She wanted him to go on in his work, but felt his studies were breaking up the family. I asked him why he did not work alone, in the front room. He replied that he liked to be with the family. I pointed out that he was poor company while he was studying, and that he would be better able to concentrate on his own. I suggested he divided his off time into hours of study on his own, and leisure hours with the family when he joined the family circle heart and soul. I asked him if he resented my intrusion into his family problems. He assured me he was not in the least upset and that I had shown him things in a new light. When I saw Mrs. L. a few weeks later she told me things were now much better.

In the same way Mrs. N.J. came to see me with vague complaints. After a while she told me her husband was not satisfied with her and that he grumbled too much. The house and the children were never clean enough for him. Sexually they appeared compatible. He was very generous and sensible with her as regards his pay, but he was always grousing. I asked to see her husband. I told him I had discussed certain things with his wife and before reaching the point of difference between the two, told him how sensible he was about his pay and praised all possible points of argument. Having told him his wife felt upset because he was not satisfied with her standard of housekeeping, he remarked that she was very different from his mother. He then amazed me by saying how it upset him to run his handkerchief along the picture rail and find dust on it. I told him if he was as critical as all that, I did not wonder at his wife's resentment. I suggested that while he was the master of his own job and his wife had to fit her life round his work, so she was the mistress of the house, and how she ran it was more her business than his. I suggested criticism rarely stirred anyone to action, whereas praise for good work was far more encouraging. When I saw him later he told me things were much better. He recounted how on one occasion he found his wife tidying out a cupboard and he had congratulated her on her efforts. He felt she was trying to keep up a better standard and he evidently was less critical.

All marital differences are not settled so easily ; and there are many hopeless cases where intervention by a third party is too late to be effective, but an attempt at mediation can do little harm and there is often a chance of doing good. In actual practice one is rarely asked to mediate in a hopeless case, for help, if sought at all, is usually asked for before the trouble has gone too far, and it is quite amazing what simple troubles can appear insolvable to the partners in such an intimate and emotional contract as marriage. No very profound wisdom or superhuman intelligence is required of the practitioner who is asked to solve these problems but merely the perspective which comes of detachment from the emotional situation. Every general practitioner who views himself as a family doctor and not as a clerk signing certificates and directing his patients to specialists should be willing to undertake this form of treatment when required, for if he succeeds he allays not only the anxiety of the pair immediately involved but also of all the members of the family unit.

REFERENCES

(i) D. R. MACE. Marriage Crisis. 1948.

(ii) G. DICK READ. Antenatal and Postnatal Care, by F. J. Brown. 1942.

(iii) E. F. GRIFFITH. Modern Trends in Psychological Medicine. 1948.

CHAPTER XIII

THE FUTURE OF PSYCHIATRY

Most general practitioners are content to leave the future of psychiatry to the psychiatrist. The treatment of mental illness is, however, seen from very different view points by the family doctor on the one hand and the alienist on the other, and it is because of this great difference that I venture as a general practitioner to speculate on the future.

The experts live in an atmosphere of mental hospitals, in a world in which institutional treatment of mental illness is an accepted fact, and therefore methods of improving the treatment are their chief aim. They labour at present under great difficulties, with shortages of staff, buildings and equipment, shortages indeed of everything except patients; in such circumstances their view of the future tends to be distorted by the present overwhelming difficulties. Their chief concerns are with the treatment of their patients who have arrived at the mental hospital, and with the eradication of administrative difficulties. The general practitioner is confronted with a very different side of the picture. He is faced with a family unit in which mental illness has been diagnosed in one of its members. The suggestion of a mental hospital prostrates the whole family. The patient does not want to go and the relatives do not want to send him. In the early stages of disease when help would be most beneficial, they affirm he is not bad enough, and so they wait until the disease has a firmer hold. He can only be sent away when the family doctor has the whole family behind him, unless of course the patient is a danger to himself or others. The responsibility is considerable. The certification of a patient suffering from paranoia, who may be normal in every respect apart from his monomania, may be equivalent to a life sentence, and, unlike the High Court judge, the general practitioner has no jury to decide a verdict. Certification is a serious decision for the practitioner and a calamity for the family unit. Once the patient is in a mental hospital the whole family feels stigmatised and even if the victim is a voluntary patient, it makes very little difference. At best the patient recovers, and everyone tries to forget the incident. At worst the patient does not recover and the family blame the mental hospital atmosphere. They argue that the patient could hardly be expected to recover surrounded by such strange cases. The history of mental illness in a family is always most difficult to extract. It is often emphatically denied and one hears the true story from other sources. The problem is even more difficult when one is faced with a patient who is not insane, but who needs treatment which can only be obtained in a mental hospital. One may have spent a lot of time reassuring an obsessional or a neurotic that he is not suffering from a mental illness and that fears of insanity are without foundation, and then one has as a last resort to suggest a mental hospital for treatment. It is grievous when the victim of a severe neurosis prefers to put up with a crippling neurotic illness rather than face a mental hospital, and when rapport, built up over hours of work, is broken completely by the suggestion. Once a neurotic patient has acquired a negative transference towards psychiatry and psychiatrists of all kinds, it is difficult if not impossible to woo him back to radical treatment.

The following statement was made by a mild depressive who had been persuaded to go into a mental hospital. His exact words are quoted.

"As a voluntary patient for a short time in a mental home, I would like to state my opinion. I went to the home suffering from depression. Well, in the first place I must say I disagree with sending patients with the same complaint as myself to a mental home. I will not say all, but quite a few get more depressed than ever after being in the hospital for a week or so, and they have very good reason for being so. I will tell you how I felt myself. In the first place I was sent to bed for two weeks as the doctor said I needed complete rest. But how could one rest when the poor fellows who were certified lunatics in another part were shouting and making a horrible noise, both day and night? It was impossible to rest. When I was allowed to get up and walk about I could not help meeting some of them. I felt sorry for them but at the same time it made me feel more depressed than ever. I wasn't having any treatment of any kind, and when I asked the doctor about it, he told me that being in the home was treatment. By now, having very little sleep and meeting those poor fellows my only thought was to get away from the home.

"Then there is another point and a big one in my opinion. I should like to say this as the patient in the next bed expressed it to me. He turned to me one day and told me this story. He was single but engaged to be married. He had not told his girl which hospital he had gone in, simply because he did not want her to know he had gone to a mental home. So while he was there, he had no letters from his girl friend. He asked me this, 'Why have I come here? I know I am depressed and I feel horribly low in myself, but I am not insane. Why should I come here to a place like this, which I must if I want to get better, because this is the only place I can get treatment for this complaint. I am sane, so why should I be sent to a lunatic asylum?' There were tears in his eyes as he said this, but I could not answer him, because I had thought the same things myself.

"As a voluntary patient you can leave the hospital if you give them 72 hours' notice and I am afraid there are quite a few patients hand in their notice before they are really well, because they don't like being in a lunatic asylum. So I hope with all my heart that in the near future fellows who have the same complaint as I had will not have to go to a lunatic asylum or a mental hospital which is more or less the same thing, to get better again. Sooner have a hospital which deals only with this sort of complaint so that a fellow does not lose his self respect with the thought that he was once a patient in a lunatic asylum, even though he was sane."

A patient in this state of mind will not readily return for treatment at the first sign of a relapse although he appreciates fully that, as he says, it is the only place where he can get treatment for his complaint ; nor would he advise any friend to follow such a course with any kind of cheerful confidence. A great many man-working days are lost before treatment is sought, and recovery is made more difficult through the reluctance and added depression associated with the final decision that such treatment must be accepted.

It is many years since the serious nature of venereal disease in the life of the nation made itself felt. Lock hospitals were opened but they were not the complete answer. The treatment had to be secret and confidential and patients were loath to visit hospitals which advertised their condition by the very fact of the visit. Because of this in many places departments were opened at general hospitals so that patients could be afforded a cloak to cover their complaint. Thus no stigma was attached to their visits, and progress was made in combating these diseases. It seems reasonable to suppose that if a similar arrangement could be made for the benefit of psychiatric patients, neuroses and psychoses would more readily accept treatment in their early stages. The use of the term mental hospital instead of lunatic asylum has done something to help the public to adopt a more rational attitude towards such institutions but as long as any institution caters only for neurotic and psychotic conditions it remains branded in the eyes of the general public. An excellent hospital such as the Crichton Royal, is a kind of Mecca in the eyes of all medical men who are interested in psychiatry, but even it fills the average patient with foreboding. "I would rather die than go there" one depressive told me with great feeling. Of course there are patients big enough to accept the hospital as they accept their illness, but such are the exception rather than the rule. It takes a great deal of courage to let the doors of a mental hospital close behind you however attractive the flowers in the lobby may be. It is my experience that very few will do it until certification becomes a painful necessity. If patients could slip unobtrusively into a general hospital few would object, but it will take a great deal of skilled propaganda to make the man in the street view a mental hospital with anything but fear and distrust. Once inside its walls he tends to feel he will never get out again. If it is not too difficult to make arrangements which make it easy for patients suffering from venereal disease to seek treatment, surely it should not be impossible to be equally considerate towards the victims of nervous and mental illness. To effect such a change would, of course, involve a tremendous capital outlay, but once established, its working would be so much more economical than the present system that ultimately the initial cost would be worked off. Each large general hospital would need its neuropsychiatric wing with open and closed wards and centres for psychotherapy, occupational therapy and all special forms of treatment. The severe depressive or early schizophrenic patient would be referred to the general hospital. Here he would be seen by the specialist and admitted to the appropriate ward. The severe depressive would have to be kept under careful observation in the closed ward at first. With treatment the crisis of his depression would be passed in a few weeks and the patient would then be transferred to an open ward for a period, with full freedom of the hospital facilities before his discharge. He would probably not be off work for more than four to six weeks, and he would have no hesitation in returning for a repeat of the treatment should he break down again. He would return home having been at the "City General" for observation and treatment. At worst his neighbours would regard him as "one of those nerve cases"; the question of lunacy, madness, or insanity would never arise.

The schizophrenic would follow a similar course with a routine insulin therapy or more advanced discoveries in substitution therapy. Some would recover and be discharged through the open ward, but many would degenerate into the typical hopeless case and would then have to be removed from the closed wards to make room for other patients more likely to benefit from the treatment. If such a patient were amenable and had relatives who were willing and able to look after him he could be sent home as other incurables are sent home when the hospital can do no more for them. If he were too bad to be sent home or had no suitable home to which to go, then and then only he would have to be certified and sent to a mental hospital. Temporary certification might well be necessary in order to send an acute or violent case to hospital against his will, but he should still be able to be sent to the general hospital where he would be admitted to the closed ward and treated as an emergency, and most of them would recover and be able to be discharged later. Mental hospital statistics show that today, with modern methods of treatment, about 70 per cent of admissions are discharged as recovered or improved. It seems a pity that so many people should be stigmatised, when they could have been treated as well in a properly equipped general hospital.

The vast majority of neurotics and mild depressives should be treated as out patients, receiving their treatment weekly or twice weekly, some remaining at work in the meantime. Where hospitalisation was necessary for intensive treatment the patient would be admitted to an open ward and would never be confronted with the mentally deranged inhabitants of the closed wards any more than an asthmatic would be confronted with views of the operating theatre, the labour ward, or the mortuary.

Every nurse should have mental nursing included in her curriculum. Thanks largely to this omission from training, the functional cases are frequently misunderstood and despised by sisters and nurses as a whole. Neurotics are, in their estimation, feeble creatures full of imaginary complaints, while psychotics are feared and are ejected from any respectable ward with all possible speed. The welfare of the patients is sometimes forgotten in the haste to dispose of them. The period of time served by probationer nurses in the neuro-psychiatric wards would add considerably to the value of their training, and if the attitude of the V.A.D.'s in the last war is any criterion they would be very interested in the work. The care of acute psychiatric cases is as intricate and absorbing as anything in medicine. The psychiatric wing would be a cheerful and progressive place in which the atmosphere would be free of all the gloomy dread which must retard the progress of many patients in mental institutions today. Patients would come earlier for treatment and there would be far fewer serious and incurable cases than there are today to be transferred to mental hospitals. The mental hospitals for incurables could easily be superintended by an intelligent layman with supervision from the medical staff of the local general hospital. The nursing in these hospitals would be very dull and staff would have to be attracted by special rates of pay. The whole scheme would however absorb far less professional time than the present day system and the rise in the recovery rate would save immense numbers of man-working days and the money saved for the nation would more than pay for the expense of any such scheme.

Until the discovery of new and effective physical methods of treatment, combined with adequate psychotherapy, the mental hospital was merely a sanctuary for the mentally disordered. They were protected and cared for until remission set in. If there was no remission they were inmates for life. While such conditions obtained, it was clearly impossible to incorporate a neuropsychiatric wing into a general hospital except for the treatment of neuroses. The advent of new and better methods of treatment has now made such a change possible, and indeed desirable, if the problem is going to be solved in a reasonable space of time. Propaganda may remove the stigma from a mental hospital in a century or more, but to try and pretend that today there is no deterring stigma is about as futile as reassuring a child with a painful dressing, that the doctor won't hurt.

With such a system many of our present day mental hospitals would not be required. They need not be wasted. In the future many prisons will give way to psychopathic hospitals and the remote, barred, prison-like buildings which house our mental patients today could be admirably adapted for this purpose. In Denmark this system is already in practice. The antisocial psychopath is not given a prison sentence; he is referred to a psychopathic hospital where he stays until he can prove to the authorities by his behaviour and his power of work that he is fit for freedom and the privileges of citizenship. His sentence is indeterminate, and unless he can reform and prove himself able to master his emotions, his sentence is for life. Fifty per cent of these criminal psychopaths get discharged and few thereafter relapse. This is surely a wiser process than the limited sentence imposed by our law; whereby psychopaths go to prison and are released after serving their sentence only to commit more crimes (i).

In the future some kind of hospitalisation might well be extended from criminal psychopaths to hysterics. It is axiomatic in psychiatry and general medicine that illness must not be made profitable for the patient. In the present system of social security illness is indeed made profitable for some hysterics and there is little hope of curing them on that account. Most of us have a few incurable hysterics on our lists who haunt our surgeries, and who can live comfortably at home on the club without doing a stroke of work to support themselves or their families. Psychotherapy will not help them. They are immature people who need kindly but firm discipline. There is real efficacy in a bucket of cold water actual or metaphorical but it is difficult to administer in the home, and rarely increases the popularity of one's practice. A spell in an institution can sometimes carry out a duty which no general practitioner could perform.

Firm, sympathetic and impersonal discipline can often work wonders if the patient is detached from fawning relations who are all too willing to be over sympathetic to him.

In all branches of medicine present and future, systems of hospitalisation are a superstructive which have to be built upon a foundation provided by general practitioners. If general practitioners accept the roll of clerks or sign posts directing their patients to the appropriate out-patient department, those departments will become so overcrowded that the whole system will break down. To make the work of the out-patient department of the psychoneurotic wing possible, patients must only be sent there after they have been dealt with rationally by their general practitioners. Not every doctor possesses an interest in psychiatry. Some will wish to avoid it as others avoid midwifery, and in the future one must therefore envisage the general practitioner psychiatrist just as there is a general practitioner obstetrician today. It may well be that the tripod of medicine will become a tetrapod and the youngest branch of medicine will be represented by the Royal College of Psychiatry, and like the present Royal College of Obstetricians the new college will cater for the general practitioner as well as the consultants and offer some suitable qualification. Every group practice would see to it that one of its members was a general practitioner psychiatrist and to him would drift the majority of the psychotic and neurotic cases in the practice but only as an integral part of his general work. He would remain essentially a general practitioner from the patient's point of view, as likely to handle midwifery or appendicitis as "nerves". Psychiatric work takes up more time that the average case so that he would have to be allowed more time for special consultations than his colleagues, but it would be most undesirable for him to aim at being a full time psychiatrist. He must remain essentially a jack of all trades, for it is his capacity to tackle all and sundry that develops his special powers of judgment and gives him his peculiar knowledge of his patients and their background. The general practitioner psychiatrist must be first and foremost a general practitioner with a secondary interest in, or bias towards psychiatry. The bulk of psychiatric work inevitably falls to the general practitioner, and unless more encouragement is given for such work the problem will never receive the attention it deserves. General practitioners as a whole must undertake their full share of the work, and the complacent dispensing of placebos must be superseded by simple but radical psychotherapy.

With such general practitioners distributed throughout group practices, 80–90 per cent of cases would be dealt with entirely in the general practitioner's consulting room. The remaining 10–20 per cent would be referred to consultants and half would require out patient treatment, the remaining half being admitted to hospital. Of these admissions about 1 per cent would become chronic and require certification and transfer to the mental institutions.

Such a system would be economical and efficient in the treatment of psycho-neurotic cases. But prevention is better than cure and psychology is not the peculiar province of the physician. Medical psychology is only one branch of the subject and it is the reparative rather than the preventative branch. School and industrial psychologists will do much in the future to ease the burden that today falls on the general practitioner. When casualties have occurred and need to be referred to neuro-psychiatric departments much of the psychotherapy could be done by lay psychologists. The problem is so great that the medical profession can never hope to solve it alone.

Many mental hospitals, as they are today, are obsolete. Let only the hopeless and incurable cases, and the psychopaths be relegated to such institutions, where the confinement and the control serves a useful purpose and are not an unfortunate deterrent to those who most need help. Most neurotics and psychotics are worthy of greater consideration. Mental disease is more terrifying than most of our human troubles. Surely it is high time we took steps in a big way to make the prevention and treatment of such troubles as easy and pleasant for the patient as possible, by removing from our midst the bogey of the mental hospital and the associated stigma. When the authorities realise this and plan to enlarge our general hospitals to treat psychiatric cases, then indeed the lot of the patient and work of both the general practitioner and the psychiatrist will be made so much easier and more pleasant.

REFERENCE

(i) S. TAYLOR. Lancet, 1949, i, **32**.

INDEX